HOME BIRTH

A Modern Memoir on Pregnancy, Midwives, Fitness and Choices

I0022263

by
Cera Gagnon

Foreword by
Rachel Sutton, Midwife

CCB Publishing
British Columbia, Canada

Home Birth: A Modern Memoir on Pregnancy,
Midwives, Fitness and Choices

Copyright ©2021 by Cera Gagnon
ISBN-13   978-1-77143-483-6
First Edition

Library and Archives Canada Cataloguing in Publication
Title: Home birth : a modern memoir on pregnancy, midwives, fitness and choices / by Cera
Gagnon ; foreword by Rachel Sutton, midwife.
Names: Gagnon, Cera, author. | Sutton, Rachel (Midwife), writer of foreword.
Description: First edition.
Identifiers: Canadiana (print) 20210241039 | Canadiana (ebook) 20210241225
| ISBN 9781771434836 (softcover) | ISBN 9781771434843 (PDF)
Subjects: LCSH: Gagnon, Cera. | LCSH: Pregnant women—Canada—Biography.
| LCSH: Pregnancy—Canada—Popular works.
| LCSH: Childbirth at home—Canada—Popular works.
| LCSH: Childbirth—Canada—Popular works. | LCGFT: Autobiographies.
Classification: LCC RG525 .G34 2021 | DDC 618.20092—dc23

Cover design by SelfPubBookCovers.com/Daniela

Publisher: CCB Publishing
             British Columbia, Canada
             www.ccbpublishing.com

This book is dedicated to the mothers, fathers, parents, partners, and the caregiving teams who gather together to bring babies safely and joyously into the world. To the friends, uncles, aunts and grandparents and all others who help raise and care for the young. To anyone wanting to learn more about pregnancy and birth and those who work tirelessly to share related information and empower others. To everyone who ever encouraged me along the way and told me I can, and to those who told me I can't. May we each find our unique way.

Contents

Foreword
by Rachel Sutton, Midwife

As a midwife, I have had the great privilege of witnessing the childbearing journey of hundreds of women and assisting them to bring new life into the world. I have often wished that more people had the opportunity to witness these powerful moments, which is why I am so pleased that Cera Gagnon has chosen to share her journey with the world. This book is an inspiring account of how one woman examined all her birthing options, made careful decisions, and then worked hard mentally and physically to maximize her chances of having the birth she wanted. Throughout her story Cera also helps explain the value of some lesser known birthing options such as midwives, home birth, and meditative techniques to cope with the pain of childbirth. I hope this book will inspire more pregnant women to examine all their options and feel confident in their choices.

Preface

Speaking of birth, what is an ideal birth anyways? Does it exist, somewhere in the stratospheric notions of our dreams? Do we actually know people who went through it without being scared, traumatized or scarred emotionally or physically in some way? We can apply tools and strategies for wellness in every other area of our lives to influence the outcome, so was it also possible to do the same thing when having a baby or was it all completely up to fate? Could I somehow make it through this monstrously huge transformational event with my body, my internal organs, my dignity and my spirit intact? These were the major questions I struggled with when faced with childbirth.

I suppose my overall aspirations were not that big, at least not at first. I wanted to get through it, survive it and not let it damage or become the boss of me. I wanted to come out the other side smiling, somehow! Despite the programming I received all my life, I was determined to find a way that worked and caused the least amount of harm possible to either me or my child. I wasn't fooling myself, I didn't expect to actually enjoy it or for things to be blissful. After all, it was something I had been afraid of for almost as long as I can remember. Pregnancy was also always something I would have to begrudgingly 'get through,' and seemed almost equally worth worrying about. The fear was always there, lurking behind the covers and in the corners. Even in the most open of circles we didn't seem to talk much about actually being afraid and what, if anything, we could really do about it. It would just silently loom heavy in the room. Mostly there was an unspoken 'let's hope for the best' energy with lots of head nodding and downcast eyes. Hitting this subject head-on would change me forever. It's kind of fascinating, and despite its universality it seems to remain something of a taboo, for a lot of different reasons.

I am aware that writing a book of this nature comes with a certain responsibility. When the urge to write struck I felt like an ostrich with its head in the sand. "What will everyone think? What if it comes across the wrong way?" Then I remembered the myriad of discussions I have had with other women, who have struggled in one way or another with birth and pregnancy. I cannot nor do I want to speak for other women. Each pregnant woman is unique. Just ask any willing women to share their birth stories and you will see discrepancies and variations as broad as the snowflakes are different. I have certainly swapped stories with many, many other women. I have never heard any two stories that were completely alike nor any that exactly matched my own, though a few come close. This is what makes this subject so beautiful, albeit challenging, to write about. Birth stories are tremendously personal in nature and invoke a very wide range of emotions, from pride and joy to regret and frustration, and sometimes all of these all at the same time! I sort of see pregnant women as individual ecosystems, each woman requiring different types of support and ideal conditions to flourish.

Being a little shy in my day-to-day life, writing a book of such a personal and sensitive nature was a little outside my comfort zone. I am not an expert on birth. I have experienced it three times, without drugs or fanfare, in my own special way. Despite being sanctioned legally and funded by the government in many countries, including my own, I recognize there is debate in some circles about the safety of home birth. It is not my desire, nor my intention, to open up this can of worms as the detail and complexity of analysing the data that exists is simply beyond the scope of this book. Suffice to say that plenty of information on safety and statistics is readily accessible and most midwifery groups have the research available on their websites and in their libraries, as do their governing bodies.

I was once very skeptical about birth at home and thought my birth goals completely out of reach. I changed tremendously in the process of becoming a parent. Here is my dance with fear, with the great unknown. For others who are uncertain, who may be experiencing anxiety or nervousness around birth, I offer this up as a gentle hand to hold. I have been there.

A Note on Midwifery

You might assume, perhaps, that modern women know all about the midwifery support that may be freely available to them and other tools of importance but I have repeatedly seen otherwise, myself included. The information I received changed my life along with that of my children, and I like to share it with others when I can. *Especially* with pregnant women and those who advocate for them.

For those who may be new to the topic here is a little (but far from exhaustive) overview of what the midwife as healthcare practitioner framework looks like: While home birth popularity is increasing, the vast majority of midwife deliveries still happen in hospitals and to a lesser extent at birthing centres. A midwife follows the medical model and assesses an individual's health needs and provides medical obstetric care and information throughout the length of pregnancy.

The philosophy of midwifery care centres around informed choice. Informed choice refers to having access to all relevant and available information while in a decision making process. Midwives work from the belief that pregnant women have the right to make choices about all areas of their care; that they should be given adequate information, that they should be and stay actively involved and consulted with, and that they should have plenty of opportunities and time to ask questions and to make choices.

Midwives are usually the only healthcare providers for pregnant women who offer their clients a choice of birthplace: for example, they attend births at home, in hospitals and in midwifery-led birth centres. In Ontario, Canada, midwives provide complete care as the primary care provider from early pregnancy to six weeks after delivery for both mother and baby and provide for all obstetric needs. In the case of home birth, midwives bring portable versions of emergency equipment and supplies such as suction, oxygen, intravenous fluids, tools and equipment to suture tears and medications for the prevention and treatment of postpartum hemorrhage, etc.

Typically a team of up to four midwives is assigned to one person, with one midwife acting as the primary caregiver. In most cases two midwives attend each birth. They also screen for complications and arrange consultations with physicians as required. In the event there are complications and care needs to be transferred to a physician, a midwife is usually still available for information and support if desired. They are often both funded and regulated by the government, as is the case within Canada. In many different countries worldwide midwives have various degrees of popularity and funding, (a simple Internet search will let women know what is regulated and available to them in their home areas).

Midwifery is separate from, but can be very related to, having a doula assist/attend at a birth. A doula is someone who is available before, during and beyond the birth to help a woman with a wide variety of needs, be they physical, mental or emotional. She will support a woman no matter who is her primary care provider is or wherever she decides to give birth. Whereas a midwife or physician acts as the primary care provider for the woman and baby, a doula's role is supportive in nature. She is a woman's companion whose role is to encourage, care for and comfort.

Introduction

I have a lovely friend who is rather precious to me. She likes to be helpful and encouraging and holds a healing vision for the world. Yet often, despite my best efforts to remind her of her worth, she can easily lapse back into seeking the approval of others at times. I am helping her to trust herself and her instincts, especially when big decisions role around. She is nervous and reluctant to engage in any confrontation. I know my job will take time. I am patient.

"Do you really want to look back and realize you missed the chance to publish this?"

"No, but the subject matter is way too personal, it opens me up to too much condemnation, and what if it doesn't come across as helpful?"

"You are talking about a different way to do things, a new yet old way to get through this!"

"Still. It makes me feel rather vulnerable."

"That's what taking a risk is all about, that's what leadership is all about, being vulnerable. And you are right, it is personal, but guess what? We are all persons."

I've always had this thing for knowledge. The sharing of it, the making of it available to everyone, the thirst to understand how things work and to grow my perspective, especially around the subject of health and wellness. Experienced astronaut Chris Hadfield says the more you know, the less you fear. I agree. While I dove into many topics in my youth I never touched much upon pregnancy. And why bother anyways? Almost everything I had heard about it or been exposed to on the subject was dreary and negative. I thought I would figure it out at the time. And then the time did come along. Pregnancy. Crazy cool. Seems like I had been getting ready to be a parent since I was young, taking care of my toy baby doll all day as a child, staying glued at the hip with the babies I sometimes got to babysit in my teens or cherishing every moment I possibly could with my nieces and nephews. But suddenly I had a new dilemma and big questions. I knew this was a natural process, but still, as excited as I was to be pregnant, there was also a floodgate of "what-ifs" facing me down. *How would I keep myself physically and emotionally healthy during this special period of time? How would I avoid ballooning too much in size, being emotionally overwhelmed, or having permanent physical damage? How would I manage the birth and sweet Jesus how about the pain of the birth if I tried a more natural approach?*

The baby does not technically have to move very far to go from inside to outside of the body, yet the whole process of growing a person and delivering one to the outside world seemed daunting. Giving birth was the one thing I did not want to go through, but I would have to get ready to face this reality. It was apparently going to test my physical and emotional limits to the max. At the time I would have given a fortune for someone to insist that there was a different way, or an easier way, to go through it all. Someone to squeeze my hand, and tell me things would simply be okay, that I could handle it and that I *could* influence the outcome. But I didn't have this, at least not in the beginning. This book is a journey of dealing with these obstacles and creating a path forward. It is a description of the world of becoming a parent as it appeared to me.

Like many people I know I always assumed I would end up having a baby in a hospital, as is still the general standard (though it is progressively changing, especially within the COVID stay-at-home world). When I first decided to become a parent I had a 9-5 office job, a second hand car, a small dog, and some dreams.

I vividly remember coming back to reality, slowly feeling my way out of the haze of the birth process, my youngest child in my arms as I knelt gently on the floor holding her. I remember my gentle, respectful, yet direct midwife staring at me with what I could only describe as a wistful, stunned, serious expression. She said, "Cera, whatever it is you do, what you've just done, you should teach to other women." Kind of flattered, very humbled and mostly just surprised, I thanked her and told her I might think about one day doing so, but deep down didn't think I would have the courage or energy to make it a reality.

Writing memoirs was not something I had ever really thought of until recently. During my third pregnancy I remember being in the middle of (yet another) group discussion on birth, with about 15 mostly first-time mothers standing around me chatting while they tucked their babies into carriers and car seats. They were expressing sadness and regret and complaining that each and every one of them had a negative or traumatic birth story and that 'no one at all has a positive birth story to share.' My heart broke with compassion. The last thing I wanted to do was diminish the importance of their stories or the realities they faced. I also felt like the oddball out. It seemed wise at the time to keep my very different experiences to myself. I said nothing.

Perhaps sharing my stories would not have helped those women going forward into their second pregnancies, or maybe it would have. And I would mostly keep my stories to myself for years.

Later on I realized that maybe I was wrong to continue to keep quiet with my experiences for fear it may dim the light on someone else's or for fear that someone might be taken aback that my journey was so different than theirs. My dad calls me a shy maverick. He's right about the shy part. I suppose I was also worried about ruffling the feathers of the predominant birthing regime that is in place. There are a ton of cultural underpinnings and power imbalances in our healthcare models, so raising my voice about a sometimes touchy subject seemed risky. Being fourth born, I learned early how much easier it is to stay quiet and not be noticed as much as others. But I have reached a point where it is time to make new choices. The more I researched and learned about the history of birth and how we, as a society, came to adopt the modern framework that is now in place, the more I was inspired to share my own version of events. Lack of mainstream knowledge related to wellness concerns me deeply, as does the lack of power women still sometimes experience at critical intervals in their lives.

There is a shift going on as we speak, a bit of a revolution of going 'back to the basics.' What was once seen as the only normal way to have a baby is changing, and I can testify to that. There is a huge disparity that exists in opinions and 'norms' around birth plans. I have many friends and associates now who had babies at home and who work exclusively with midwives. I also have friends and family who have never heard much about midwifery, prefer the status quo or just feel much safer in a hospital setting, and others still who think it's just plain nuts to bother going through the pain of birth on purpose and will avoid the discomfort of it as much as possible.

Everyone Has A Story

Last year one of my relatives gave birth to her first child at home very comfortably, apparently experienced little pain, fear or discomfort. I had seen her only a few months beforehand during a co-ed soccer game I hosted. She was having a ball, beating every single one of the other players, stealing the ball from anyone she pleased at five months pregnant. I have another relative with a specific chronic health condition who, after doing lots of research, decided her safest option was to book a C-section. She was able to have a midwife by her side in a supporting role, free of charge. She says she has no regrets and would do the same thing again in a heartbeat. Another woman I know used hypnobirthing as her resource of choice and sailed through her labour without any serious discomfort before, during or after. One of my favourite stories is about my best friend's grandmother, whom he described as a strong, independent and hearty woman. As the story goes, she left one early morning to go berry picking in the woods and when she arrived back home much too late that afternoon she had a basket full of berries and a baby tucked under her arm. Years ago when I first heard this story, I was impressed and yet worried and scared for her safety and emotional

1

well-being at the same time. These days I feel very differently about it.

My own mother thought she was going to die while going through her first labour (she had five natural births in total), left mostly completely alone on a hospital bed for hours (at a time when my father wasn't allowed to accompany her in the room). She describes an attending doctor who said very little to her, and the overall experience as scary and filled with uncertainty. She was given treatments in preparation for birth that were scarring and invasive without being asked first, things that were simply 'status quo' at the time. She didn't have the foresight or courage to even question how things were done. When her first baby was finally born many hours later she was moved to a new shared room. She tried in vain to request different accommodations for herself and the baby as the new mother beside her was chain smoking non-stop and she felt terrible exposing her newborn to the cloud of smoke in the room.

My grandmother's first child was born at full term, and by all accounts was robust and well developed but needed respiration support which he did not receive. There remains great controversy to this day around his death in the delivery room shortly after birth, the nurses claiming nothing was done to help him get his lungs working properly and the physician who delivered him remaining silent on the subject, except to say, 'Sorry, no baby,' to my grandmother.

These were the days when women were gassed and put to sleep to have the baby delivered. My grandma was brave but scared and did everything she was told and woke up to the unimaginable. The trauma and anguish my grandparents experienced at losing their first baby was indescribable and the legacy of this pain and powerlessness would make its way down through the family in subsequent generations both orally and emotionally, and, I think, even genetically, to some degree. If emotional trauma is indeed stored in our DNA, this one made its way down to me for sure.

Personally, when I was pregnant for the first time, I just wanted to do things as safely as possible, as quickly and easily as possible, and as comfortably as possible (in that order), and to give my body the best possible odds. Obviously I was influenced by the stories from my ancestors, but at the same time I truly had confidence that things 'had changed' in modern times and felt hopeful that maybe the hospital birthing environment would be much more welcoming and pleasant for me.

On the New Road

So many changes life brings, so many changes life sings.

The only way forward is through, just take it one step at a time.

Everything is totally new, and the only way to win is to try.

...The above represents Cera's approach to pregnancy

Can you ever really be ready to be pregnant? Probably not. I was elated. I was delighted. I was terrified. I was good enough with expecting the unknown but this was totally new territory. I read the mainstream stuff. I took a breath. I reassured myself. But yet, I was still scared. Of like, everything. As much as I was intuitively trusting the natural process of pregnancy and had faith in my body's ability, I was suddenly bombarded by doubts from all angles.

It was late autumn. I had recently moved into a new home, one I had selected virtually overnight, and I now had the space for a tree, a dog, larger indoor plants, a piano, and maybe one day even a small infrared sauna (my wish-list purchases) and certainly a baby. I was busy with a 9-5 Analyst job and two extra family members had temporarily been living with us. While I was totally stoked about the pregnancy and it was exactly what I wanted at that time, I was also suddenly anxious about all the new responsibilities on my plate (keeping myself healthy, making a birth plan, finding an obstetrician, etc.). To be honest, I was also very worried about just 'staying' pregnant. I'd had enough friends go through very brief one or two month pregnancies that terminated naturally and I was told, like most of my peers, that waiting until the three month mark to announce anything was a safer bet, 'just in case.' It's weird because what happens is that when you probably need to confide in others and receive their wisdom the most you end up keeping things to yourself instead, adding all that silence and uncertainty to the ever-growing anxiety pile.

I was also getting up at least twice during the night to potty train my puppy and the broken sleep, coupled with the changes of early pregnancy, left me feeling more tired and worn out than usual. Still, I have to say my overall attitude was 'onward and upward.' I was determined to do my best with this new role I was stepping into as a parent.

Being healthy and making sure all was on track equaled being safe for me, and I wanted to waste no time moving forward. This may have been my nerves speaking as well. I felt that as soon as I could reassure myself that things were progressing as they ought to, I would be able to breathe. As soon as I thought I was pregnant I took the steps to get booked with a female obstetrician. By the time I had my very first appointment the following month I was feeling hopeful and excited, on time, and ready to learn all I could about what to expect. I was also a little nervous and had absolutely, as in zero, idea of what to expect from the specific Obstetrician I was booking with. I am a little allergic to social media sometimes, so hadn't read testimonials or reviews before going. I planned to give birth at a hospital close to home and so my options for female doctors who worked there were limited. My plan was to have as little interference and intervention as possible and to have support from a female physician, and I was eager to meet with whoever would be on my team.

Like other women I knew, I figured I'd go meet a nice (hopefully) open-minded (maybe?) doctor who would explain the ropes and help me lovingly deliver my baby (whatever exactly 'deliver' meant I wasn't sure and was going to definitely ask about it) in as natural and peaceful a way as possible. The fear of pain was very real for me, however the risks associated with intervention were even more worrisome and I was eager to discuss these matters with my OB.

Finding Another Way

Friday afternoon after work: "I am completely at my wits end, a manager seems to have a penchant for making my life difficult at work. It is becoming harder and harder to feel any goodwill towards this person whatsoever. It's hopeless, really."

(Reiki teacher) "There is always another way or a second option. Why don't you try sending love and acceptance to the situation instead?"

"Love to this situation, to Marilyn? You have absolutely got to be kidding. I have never been more intimidated by a person. She is making my life difficult. I feel like there is nothing I can do to make things better. Sigh. Okay fine, what the heck, I'll try your advice, but I have absolutely no confidence it could help at this point."

Monday morning at work listening to announcements: "Good morning, staff. Marilyn has just been promoted and will no longer be working with you."

"!!!!!!!!!!!?????????!!!!!!!!!!!"

If I had gone into my Obstetrician's appointment with a mild curiosity about what midwifery was about, I walked out with a determination to learn at least a little more. But in all fairness I should back up a step or two. Having never really given midwifery much thought (let alone the potential of giving birth outside a hospital setting), I had followed the expected course of looking for an Obstetrician. I first went to a family clinic and talked to a very kind and open female doctor who told me that there were only one or two female obstetricians she could think of who were practicing in my end of town. She gave me a referral to one of them and wished me luck. I was feeling exhilarated and a little nervous walking into my first 'pregnancy' appointment. I felt like this was such an important thing, meeting this person who would be on my team and supporting me during one of the most crucial periods of my life. Would they 'get' me? Would I feel comfortable being totally honest and upfront with this person? Looking back now I see the naiveté there. I didn't realize the full limitations physicians are under, the need to get things done in a short amount of time, etc. It strikes me how odd it is that the system is set up in a way that somewhat prevents a relationship between patient and doctor from forming. But for this event I did not see how I could go without one. I felt I needed at least enough connection to understand the other person's values around and approach to birth. As much as we say it is only 'professional,' given the intimate nature of the role, how could it be only that?

Feeling hopeful I swallowed back some feelings of nervousness as I entered the building.

Unfortunately, while walking into this first appointment I couldn't grab onto anything that felt truly supportive. The clinic was very small and busy. The first thing that struck me was the lack of, well, celebration of birth. It felt cramped and formal. Was I, perhaps naïvely, expecting that someone would greet me somehow differently in a pregnancy clinic versus other clinics? Or that there would be even some small recognition of the sacredness of being pregnant via a picture or two of a pregnant belly on the wall? After checking in with the receptionist, I was asked to immediately step on a scale beside the entrance area. I then had about 10 minutes with a doctor who was polite, professional and seemed in a bit of a rush. I wanted to know about what the birth process would generally look like, about what I could expect, and what her approach towards birth was, which was the most important part of this relationship as far as I was concerned. All I ended up learning was that whoever was on call when I went into labour would deliver the baby (no details given on what "deliver" meant or could involve).

An ultrasound was ordered. Feeling awkward and a little uncomfortable, I asked about the safety of early monitoring and early ultrasounds and a few other standard things which were met with surprise and relatively short answers. I sensed a clear signal that a discussion on general safety wasn't welcome or necessary, at least at this juncture. I sensed that only certain questions were acceptable and worried that only some types of information would be made available to me. I was reminded of a time years ago when I had asked to know my blood type and the doctor who attended me declined, saying, "You do not need to know." I knew that I needed to work with someone who would take my questions seriously, even if the answers seemed obvious. I worried suddenly that my inquisitive nature and desire to have a woman-centred birth plan would be an annoyance, if it wasn't already.

I felt embarrassed for asking questions and felt my sense of voice rapidly diminishing, just like it had so many times before in front of people with perceived authority. What is it about these environments that makes me feel like I am not on equal ground? Why is it so hard to use my voice without feeling anxious?

At the end of our meeting the doctor congratulated me on being pregnant as she walked out the door. I appreciated the afterthought, but it was the only sense of connection I experienced in the whole encounter. I could have cried. And actually I did, more than once that day.

Of course, I know other women who have felt happy with their physicians and their whole hospital experience, and I too was hoping to 'luck out' and be assigned to someone I connected well with. Looking back, I realize my nerves and newness to the mothering role coloured and shaped my view of the situation. My discouraged reaction, I realize, had more to do with the whole model of care in place than the specific individual, who, likely, is fantastic at their job. But for my own personality, my own need to feel autonomous and safe, I would need a different way forward. I simply could not see myself being comfortable with this model of care in place, nor was the very real possibility that a complete stranger who was on-call attending to my delivery very promising.

I had the routine blood test scheduled for right after that appointment. Back then I really wasn't okay with blood tests. The blood being pulled out usually left me feeling very queasy, at best. Already feeling totally anxious about how this birth thing was going to turn out, my nervous system went into hyper-drive. Frustrated and scared, I tried to hold back tears that fell as the attendant found my vein. In one of those blood clinics where everyone sits next to everyone out in the open, I felt exposed and embarrassed for the second time in one day. I would have given anything to have had someone hold my hand and some privacy, and here I was only at the beginning of the journey.

I decided against trying to find a second obstetrician. It wasn't just about feeling emotionally safe and being in the driver seat of the birth, or even the connection to my care-provider, though those were huge considerations. Mobility concerns during labour were very real for me. I had already learned that being on your back or sitting upright leaning back is correlated with tearing. Further, I learned that doctors in my area were not allowed to deliver babies underwater; women can use the birthing tubs while under their care during labour, but they are not allowed to stay in them for the delivery of the baby. I knew I needed options that would allow me to move about freely and that being monitored or attached to equipment would only make me feel like a watched kettle. Finally, most resources I found, medical and alternative, talked about the importance of being relaxed and staying that way as much as possible while birthing. Right. Then I needed to have a new plan for birth and some new people to help me.

People around me *were* starting to spread the word about midwifery. It hadn't been my first choice so I was cautious at first, and a little skeptical. I remembered a cheerful, friendly and open-minded work colleague who had shared about her midwife experiences. She was even interviewed in a local paper and posted the article outside her office for everyone to read. I went home and got busy.

It turns out that having a midwife, including having the home birth option, is free and funded by the government. In place of a physician, a midwife would become my and my baby's primary healthcare provider until the baby was six weeks old. What I saw and read about their policies and mission made me suddenly feel right at home and the decision to accept their help was now a no-brainer for me: "Birth is seen as a normal and natural process; emphasis is on physical, emotional, mental and social health; care is provided with the least amount of intervention possible; and risks and benefits are thoroughly addressed and discussed before any decisions are made."

Having a lifelong interest in environmental issues and sustainable development, where many topics need to be addressed simultaneously to achieve any real benefit, this holistic model sat very well with me. My cautious side liked that they were available by phone 24 hours a day, 7 days a week. And when I read the following statement on their website: "Your midwife will respect you as the main decision-maker, can make recommendations about your choices and will support your decisions," I felt a great sense of relief. Maybe this would help to make it easier for me to speak up, ask questions and keep my sense of voice and personal power strong throughout this journey.

When I contacted the local team they told me they may not have room and that I would likely be put on a waiting list, but my mind was already made up that it should come to pass. And it did. I met with Mariah not long after in a bright, sunny clinic, outfitted with couches, children's toys, a small library, and private comfortable meeting rooms. Mariah was a founder of the clinic and came across as caring, welcoming and experienced. She helped me to feel at ease and we had a lengthy first appointment. I was delighted to be allowed to ask as many detailed questions as I wanted (and boy, did I ever). I asked her how many babies she had 'caught,' how many had been born at home? Under what circumstances was birth transferred to a physician, and how often did a planned home birth turn into a hospital birth? She went over all the basics with me.

I was relieved to learn that continual monitoring of heart rate and constant routine internal checks for cervical dilation during labour that are the norm under the standard model are not seen as necessary, and that midwives are trained to 'catch' (versus 'deliver') babies in any birthing position at all. I learned that transfers from home to hospital were infrequent and that most transfers happen before or in the early stages of labour for a variety of reasons, including the client simply changing their mind or being overly fatigued. Mariah told me openly about the easiest cases she'd had and the most challenging.

Mariah would see me most of the way through my first pregnancy and then another midwife was to take over towards the end, with lots of transition time. I learned that I would meet a team of midwives so that I could develop familiarity with several of them in the event they attended my birth alongside or in place of my primary midwife. This made sense to me. I was geared up to work with this team and never missed or was late for an appointment. All the necessary screening, paperwork, weigh-ins and belly measurements were done in the privacy of their nice little comfy meeting rooms (and eventually with my other children playing with the train set, toys and books close by).

When it was eventually time for the blood draws my midwives were very accommodating. They would go gently at my speed when I was ready and I was always allowed to have someone in the room with me to hold my hand. It sometimes felt more like I was going for a visit with a friendly teammate than a health appointment.

In their cozy private office space I was able to relax a little and start to feel connected to and especially develop trust in the women who would help me bring a baby into the world. They took as long as I needed during appointments and openly shared their own personal birthing experiences. It was explained to me that they were there not just to watch over me and my baby's physical health, but to be my advocate as well. They made it clear they were on my team and that all decisions would go through me.

Consistently, one by one, each midwife I met

genuinely seemed to bear no judgment on my thoughts, my weird questions or my choices. I am certain they had their individual opinions and preferences but over and over the message was: "We are here to honour you and your choices on all subjects." They certainly voiced opinions or even disagreed when needed, but I never once felt that the power over my body was out of my hands. And I was so grateful.

It was a foreign model of care I had never been exposed to and light-years away from the medical appointments I had been accustomed to. I could show any side of myself, literally and figuratively. Working with these women helped to not only normalize birth for me, but to normalize everything that came along with it: a woman's pregnant shape was celebrated, breastfeeding, nudity and placentas became matter of fact, female instincts were listened to and respected and females as warriors helping each other was status quo in this model of care. This expanded my views exponentially and allowed me to grow deeper into self-acceptance.

I certainly cannot speak for all midwives, but those on my team truly seemed to believe in the natural process of birth. I would describe them as warriors, brave for the way they have to constantly stand up to and defend their roles, even if it is in subtle ways, to families, to in-laws and spouses, and especially to the more conventional healthcare community. Even though they made sure I was (constantly it seemed!) aware of risks, I felt a steady, gentle reassurance that birth outside the conventional model was totally normal, natural and more than that, simply 'okay.'

Although I was relieved I had found a team I could easily work with, other stressors remained in place. Appointments always included talks on risks and worst case scenarios, and of course we were always manually measuring and monitoring the baby's progress. Each time everything checked out okay I breathed a sigh of relief. The whole experience of measuring my growth and becoming informed was unnerving at first, and I would head straight out to Dairy Queen after the first couple of sessions to calm my nerves. I also slightly resented having to go to these first appointments alone, but hadn't told others yet and felt guilty pushing for company which meant more time away from work. It was all so new, it reminded me of flying in a plane for the very first time, and there was so much information to take in and the birth itself to consider.

Choice of Birthplace

It is very late. Pretty quiet in the hospital except for the unknown woman sobbing loudly in the room across from us. I am sitting with a dear friend, Rosie, waiting for her baby to make its entrance. She wants as little intervention as possible. She gets uncomfortable fast. Her labour so far seems so much like one of my own. She tells us she is uncomfortable sitting down with the pressure on her sacrum. I encourage her to switch positions and she tries being upright, leaning against the back of the hospital bed. She gets comfy and things pick up even more. Rosie is handling the contractions despite their intensity and the rhythm is nice and steady. I remind her over and over she can do it, a combination of willing and pleading with her to see what I see in her. At first she disagrees with me repeatedly. "I can't do this." "Yes you can." "Oh God I can't do this." "Yes dammit you can." And then finally, I see her punch the hospital bed, hard. "I can do this." Yes. That's my girl. Rosie would like an epidural to deal with the pain, but the anesthesiologist is very busy already, and by the time he arrives it is too late in the game. She is not prepared to deal with this much pain and did not expect to go without an epidural.

Such a different environment this is. The doctor comes and goes. When it gets really intense she comes to stay. My friend is told she has to return to a sitting reclined position, that it is not possible for the doctor to

21

deliver a baby in an upright position. I have delivered twice already in this position in fact, but I bite my tongue and say nothing. My friend doesn't argue. I mentally question this move, sensing a shift in position may slow everything down, but it is clear it is not my place to object. I start to worry, I start to pray. The labour slows down almost immediately and the heart rate drops, before finally picking back up again. The baby is called 'well-behaved' now.

I encourage and try to offer comfort as Rosie suffers and struggles a great deal to bring her baby into the world. Things continue to progress at a slower rate. My heart is in my throat. Oh God. This has to end well. I am terrified and a cold determination takes hold. If I ever, ever threw out more healing energy to a situation in my life it was then. I was not going to take this lying down. I am here, and if all l can do to help is to lend my struggling friend every single ounce of willpower that I have then so be it.

After many nerve-wracking moments of uncertainty the baby is finally born. My friend is very courageous. I try to help in any way I possibly can. The baby is placed on a table for what feels like way too long. Her fear and constant crying is very challenging for me, my instinct to hold her or at least take her hand while they take her blood pressure and cut her chord is overwhelming me. My friend cannot leave the bed. I say nothing. I eventually help Rosie into a more comfortable position for nursing. My friend is still crying and very much in pain when I have to leave. A lot of damage occurred during birth and the 'repair work' is being done. I am really not ready to go. This has been eye-opening. This has been the greatest gift. I am humbled. I am awed. I am grateful. I am unnerved and confused. I am sad. I say nothing.

I did not go into this experience having much knowledge of 'home birth' beyond hearing that someone knew someone who might have been the hippie-type living somewhere in the states had practiced it, and of course the occasional media story about a baby being born by accident in a car or what have you. I also knew that my maternal Irish/Scottish/Canadian grandmother was born at home about 100 years ago, and her mother, a nurse, acted as an unofficial local volunteer midwife and went to other women's homes to help them deliver their babies. But that was all before births became routinely hospitalized in their area. It wasn't until I met with my midwife team that I even considered the idea. I was not really open to it at first to be honest. I was biased and my beliefs about it defaulted to the cautious side. Despite a desire for a natural and non-medicated birth, I, along with most people I knew at the time, thought that the whole idea of a home birth simply 'sounded sketchy.'

It wasn't that I was completely closed to the concept per say, it's just that I bought into the common dogma that says 'births happen at hospitals,' 'pregnancy is a medical condition requiring medical attention,' and that any birth outside a hospital is 'dangerous' or even 'crazy.' There just seemed plenty to worry about as it was, why would you take that extra risk on purpose?

No one I knew personally at that point had given birth outside of a hospital. Working with a midwife as a primary care provider instead of an obstetrician was still somewhat "out there," but actually having a baby at home, *on purpose*? Wasn't that taking things too far? My mindset would change at this point. So much programmed dogma had snuck in without me realizing it.

Talk about a lesson in leaving my judgments at the door and having my opinions turned on their head. I went from thinking it was sketchy and dangerous to being convinced it was the safest option, for me personally that is. As previously mentioned, pregnant women in Ontario, Canada under the care of a midwife get to choose where to give birth. The idea that a birthplace could actually be a choice I made was rather, well, exciting and liberating to me. Suddenly new doors opened up and I was free to explore different options. My safety and that of the baby has always been paramount for me. And that definitely includes physical and emotional and mental safety. I see myself and all women who are pregnant more like an ecosystem than just a body. I looked at finding and choosing a birth location from this lens: Where was I personally going to be and *feel* the most secure, where was I able to move about, stretch or be in water? Where would I be able to be most present to do my best? This was an informed decision making process and it was *very* gradual.

My first attempt at a birth plan involved hoping to find a nearby hospital that was as private and cozy as possible. I am not sure if other people give as much thought or attention to the actual physical space they will birth in but for me this was absolutely relevant. Since I knew I needed to feel emotionally okay to be physically okay, I searched out a physical birthing space that could accommodate that. I wasn't really feeling the vibe when I saw the hospital birthing spaces. I felt a lack of warmth and privacy in many of them, and was worried I wouldn't be able to get into a comfortable 'zone' in them. I was also concerned about a host of other things. I didn't know if I'd be most comfortable birthing while standing or kneeling or leaning forward or being in a birthing tub or what, but I knew I needed a place that would afford me a good deal of options.

My next choice at the time would have been to consider the birthing centres that are now available in Ontario. This seemed like a possible option. They are set up more like a home environment with music, coziness, privacy, couches, private bathroom, etc. There is an ambulance on standby and the hospital is nearby if required. However the local birthing centre, while fully equipped, wouldn't be officially opening until the following year. So I had two choices, neither one overly appealing. A hospital within my jurisdiction or at home. *At home.* The idea still seemed wild. I kept having discussions with the midwives. Gradually, one by one, my major concerns were addressed and I started leaning towards making this a reality.

It took some time to really make up my mind, and even then I had back up plans (just in case). I registered at two local hospitals (as is common practice) in the event I changed my mind or needed to be admitted before or during labour for any reason and we made sure that distance and travel times were well laid out. By the time my third trimester rolled around I had more officially decided to proceed with having the baby at home. When it was explained to me that the midwives would check in with me in the days leading up to, the day of, and would stay with me throughout labour, I felt even more comfortable with the decision. They gave us a list of some supplies we might need such as receiving blankets, a tarp, flashlights, a sealed container (for the placenta), etc., and we kept a big box of everything and more that was needed ready to go.

PMS *While* Running A Marathon?

Another awkward moment. Another should I or shouldn't I share? Well it's a good thing I have plenty of experience feeling like the un-cool one. I listen attentively as a pregnant friend shares her fears about tearing, stitches, and long-term internal consequences.

"OMG hell no I have never heard about that, (loud mocking laughter) are you completely kidding me? You are not serious, Cera, are you?"

"No guys, it's for real. The midwives gave me a printed handout about it. It says here …the oil helps condition and soften the tissues and the massage itself helps gently stretch the area to lessen potential tearing and long-term tissue and nerve damage."

"Um, yeah, nope, that's crazy, (more laughter) oh geez, I would never… as if you are even talking about this…"

"Ha ha, okay wait guys, stop laughing at her, this is a real thing, I actually have heard of it too, but like, I would never do it or anything."

When people ask me about my story or any health topic I used to share enthusiastically, and this would generally go one of two ways (see above). But now I prefer to urge others to do their homework, to check the variety of sources on a topic for themselves. The thing is, like myself, I find a lot of people do not realize they *have* a variety of options when it comes to their pregnancy plans and health appointments *every single step of the way*. I had to learn about and weigh the pros and cons for many screening procedures and tests while I was pregnant and it was very eye-opening. Somehow I just didn't realize I could refuse or accept any of the things that were on the table. *"Okay, what is that test for, what are the statistics, what is my actual risk, what is the benefit and does it outweigh the short-term and long-term side effects of these procedures?"*

It was empowering to be in the driver's seat of my own health, yet it put more responsibility and pressure on my shoulders. These were decisions that I previously would have put in the hands of others and now we were deciding things as a team. I had to really talk to other women, find different kinds of birth stories, watch helpful videos and research a great deal to get a sense of what would work for *me and my pregnancy*. It was beyond eye-opening. Those pregnancy months involved learning, watching, interviewing, questioning and meditating on all sorts of birth-related opinions, science, testimonials and viewpoints. Some information was contradictory (for example: *don't do Kegel exercises because it will tighten your passage when pregnant, versus absolutely do them because they will strengthen your birthing muscles*). Some of the routine things women underwent were too risky for my taste and I wanted to find a way to do things that simply made the most logical sense to me. There must be some way to increase my odds of having an uncomplicated, scarring delivery. Turns out there was.

I learned a lot about the importance of moving often and staying flexible and about not sitting for long periods of time, especially in the 'bucket seat' position to help the baby into and to stay in the best possible position. I started sitting on the edge of my chairs and just sitting in yogi pose with my legs crossed on the floor as much as possible. I also borrowed a non-gravity chair and a yoga ball for my office at work and I would alternate between them every hour or so, or I would just stand. People would raise the odd eyebrow when they saw me sitting on the floor at work. Oh well. To help my circulation and avoid putting pressure on my veins, I spent at least fifteen minutes each evening lying down with my legs stacked up against a wall while I read a book or did some visualization exercises. Issues with veins run in the family so as an added precaution I also massaged my legs with sesame oil each day doing upward strokes toward the heart. My swollen by the end of the day feet and legs loved it and it was nice to feel like I was taking care of myself.

Then there was the part about the pain and the need for privacy during labour to consider. This is really the big fat elephant in the room. Most people I speak with don't get an exception from either. I was hoping and praying that I would be one of the lucky ones who went through it easily with little pain, yet I intuitively sensed I would not.

I was very interested in natural pain management methods. I scoured the Internet and libraries for any source of information I could find. Practicing increasing pain tolerance by putting ice cubes on the skin, using a TENS (transcutaneous electrical nerve stimulation) unit, water birth, shower birth, massage, acupressure, you name it I looked into it.

In my second pregnancy I followed up on a suggestion from my eldest sister and found my way to hypnobirthing. I had a toddler to take care of so I could only squeeze in the self-hypnosis sessions about once a week. I would listen to the self-hypnotizing instructional CD after meditation and pranayama and let it soothe me (and it usually even put me to sleep).

The one thing I felt would be right, all three times we went through the birth process, was to have a nice birthing tub filled up with warm water available for use. I visualized how comforting and soothing it would be to sit and soak and let the water support me through the delivery. For the first two home births we booked nice little portable tubs you can fill with warm water. They tend to be popular and you have to sign up on a waiting list to rent one. We brought them home, had everything set up and ensured the space around the tub was tidy and welcoming.

I walked into a cousin's house during my early pregnancy ready to share my happy news with my extended family. Why was I so nervous at the same time? It took me awhile to make my announcement, feeling certain my exhilaration, joy and worries were all reflected in my eyes and expression. One person got up immediately, gave me a hug and said congratulations. That felt nice. Someone else said, 'Oh cool,' and a third person said loudly, "*One word: Epidural!*" Awkward silence. Um, thank you?

You know, I agree that the body is like a temple and I am all about loving it and taking good care of it as best we can. But I'm not a Martyr. I do my very best to deal with pain but ultimately am bothered and discouraged by pain as much as anyone else. I have been through plenty of situations where I wouldn't have been able to function without pain medication. Regarding medicated birth, however, I was surprised by the list of risks and consequences of epidurals for mom and baby, which just seemed to go on and on, and included additional intervention, slowing down labour and lack of mobility.

The only consistent analogies that had been given to me were that birth was like 'running a marathon' and that the labour pains were 'like the worst period cramp ever, times about 50.' Okay then. With that starting point, I could at least relate on a tiny level. I have not done a marathon or even a half-marathon but I had done various long distance races and had been running regularly for many years. I knew what helped in that arena. Building endurance, muscle strength I could rely on, pacing myself, eating lightly beforehand, being rested, stretching my muscles after exertion, staying focused and breathing consciously.

The more tricky part with my analogy puzzle was how in the heck do I prepare myself for a bad period cramp times about 50? Lucky for me, I had a nice long history of very, very painful cramps. And I am not exaggerating here. For years and years I had been working on reducing the pain naturally without the constant use of over-the-counter drugs that tended to give me indigestion and make me tired the next day. I had developed some tools and methods that seemed to help me get through the pain *if* I had the luxury of staying at home in peace with no major outside commitments. *But,* if I had to go to work or to an event or had a major paper to write, then out came the Advil. To go through the discomfort without medicating myself substantially I really, *really* had to be relaxed and present.

The only place I wanted to be with seriously painful stomach cramps was at home alone snuggled in my room with a comfortable blanket.

Being in warm water and moving my body through very gentle poses, including hip openers and supported hands and knees pose (tabletop) had helped me in the past, as did non-inflammatory easy to digest foods, lots of water and tea, and just staying calm, totally calm. I remembered that when I was tense my uterine muscles would automatically contract and make the cramping much worse. I also remembered how, occasionally when the weather was nice and time permitted, I would go for long *slow* walks. Very contemplatively, gently putting one foot in front of another, for long periods of time. If I stayed with a very slow and gentle pace my discomfort would be quite manageable.

I also thought a lot about Ina May Gaskin's *Sphincter Law* anecdotes. The sphincter law is the idea that most women need privacy in order for a sphincter, including the cervix, to open and dilate. Her documented experiences working with many birthing women showed their dilation progress would slow when they were interrupted by strangers entering the birth room or when they felt shy or embarrassed. Oh yes. That sounded like me. So where was I going to be most physically comfortable? Who did I want around me? How would I say no to the others? How would I keep my spirits high and stay positive even though I was likely to be very, very scared? I agonized over some of these questions my first time around as a mother.

Emotional safety, for me, was highly linked to my physical safety and I just could not separate them.

Finally there were plenty of other, more, ahem, delicate matters to consider. For starters, circulation issues run in the family and I needed to take my vein health seriously. I also saw all around me women who suffered long-term damage to the pelvic floor and urinary system that affected their quality of life in all sorts of limiting ways. Finding out information on the basic problems was easy enough, but finding out how to *prevent* or *avoid* things like varicose veins, hemorrhoids, long-term damage to the "elimination system," incontinence and uterine prolapse, was easier said than done. Some information came from doctors who had written books, some came by word of mouth. I learned about the power of position during labour in taking pressure off the rectum and urinary muscles. I learned about pelvic floor physio before and after to treat torn vaginal tissue and about keeping inflammation in all pelvic floor tissues low through diet. Bit by bit I pieced it all together, learning as best I could beforehand versus after the fact.

Resources, Support, *aaaand...* Cindy Crawford??

I am so very tired today. Unusually so. I even feel the need to lie down in the office and see if I can rest. What on earth is going on? Why are my eyes slamming shut? I know I am apparently supposed to be tired when pregnant but this is overboard. Is this normal or is there something I am missing?

My midwife called me later that afternoon. Everything made immediate sense. My blood test showed very low iron levels. I had to bring them up immediately and only had just over a month before my due date.

"What? Okay wow that makes sense. What is the fastest way to do this? Stop for chicken nuggets on the way home?"

"You don't have to start eating meat. You could just start taking Floravit (liquid plant-based iron) in small amounts several times a day."

"I have been taking it, well ok not every day I suppose."

"Your baby will leech every nutrient it possibly can from your body. You have to take your nutrition intake very seriously these last months."

"Gotcha."

I believe knowledge is power. I am talking about all types of knowledge: scientific, personal perspectives and anecdotes, and oral histories. I learned a great deal on my path to motherhood. The most helpful of the resources I found were discussions with other women and my midwives along with their well-stocked libraries and websites.

There were also helpful books and I feel that some are worth mentioning:

Bountiful, Beautiful, Blissful by Gurmukh is an encouraging and practical, women-centred guide to pregnancy and birth that is infused with tips taken from kundalini yoga. It includes a rather moving overview of the author's own hospital and at-home birth experiences.

Ina May's Guide to Childbirth was invaluable for me. Ina is one of the more famous midwives in North America. This is an encouraging, down-to-earth, descriptive, no-holds-barred guide to pregnancy and birth and includes lots of practical tips, resources, research and reassurances for moms-to-be.

Orgasmic Birth by Elizabeth Davis and Debra Pascali-Bonaro is empowering, unique and calls on women to tap into their natural, instinctive selves. I found this was a great one to have my hubby read. I think it explained certain perspectives better than I could at the time. There is also an inspiring video that is based on the book which is easily accessible online.

There were also other resources I used, reaching into my own memory banks I found a treasure or two...

Over twenty years ago, I wouldn't really have associated a supermodel known to all with promoting home birth or sharing a home birth story in detail. As it happened one day I was waiting for someone while they attended an appointment in a health clinic and decided to peruse a health magazine to pass the time. I came upon an article by Cindy Crawford. That's interesting, I thought. I knew of her only up to that point in time as the lovely model who had been very successful. But this wasn't a fashion magazine or even a celebrity magazine. I am not someone to focus on fashion, style or anything even really close to the world of supermodels. But this article was different. Even years before I would be ready to consider getting pregnant, Cindy was sharing her birth story. Out loud and publicly. And not just that, it was *a midwife-supported at-home birth story*! Now this was intriguing.

I had never read or heard anything like her story. It was honest, real, and relatable. It was empowering and inspiring to see her relate the details of her experience, how she felt before, during and after, overcame her fear and made it through the challenging painful moments with her midwife and husband by her side. This was not something she thought she would ever do until going to a pre-natal yoga class earlier in her pregnancy. (This was pre-yoga for me, so little did I know how much my own story would one day reflect the one I was reading at the time).

The biggest thing that struck me was the perception shift this article created in me. Here is a famous mainstream woman finding her way through natural childbirth, at home, and happily reaching out to help other women by sharing her story. Touched deeply by the article, I tucked the inspiring story away in the back of my mind for many years.

Another important resource for me was birth videos and documentaries. The value that I received from watching various home birth videos was truly priceless. I am deeply and forever grateful to all the brave women around the world who shared their personal journey on film so that people like me could get acclimatized and learn first-hand about the whole ordeal. Midwife centres typically have videos available that clients can borrow (this is where I found mine) and there are also plenty of tactful, moving documentary videos online. I watched at least twelve home birth films, from beginning of labour to end, and bawled my eyes out each and every time. By the time the video ended, baby in arms, I felt I knew or was somehow connected to the mother and family members and caregivers present. The beautiful part of watching home birth or midwife-supported birth is that they are all very unique and show you a variety of different possibilities. For example, private births, family births, births outside in the back yard in nature, births in the shower or tub, births standing, births in bed, a variety of birthing positions, births that end up being transferred to a hospital, and so forth.

At first watching birth videos was a little nerve wracking but gradually I began to see them with a sense of 'normalcy.' It helped me to see it as just a natural, deeply moving and beautiful process. Most of the documentaries openly depicted the true levels of discomfort, pain and fear the mother was going through. I was very inspired and reassured that these women were able to go through sometimes very painful births naturally, to face their fears, with no medication, and that they came out mostly smiling on the other side. It was also cool to see babies that were calm, peaceful and alert as they started on their journeys.

Home Birth

Pregnancy, for Fitness Sake

"I used to do the same thing you do."

"Come again?"

"You know, sweating and dancing and being active."

Silence

"Well I wanted to warn you that my baby girl turned out to be very alert, very awake, and had a hard time being put to asleep. So I avoided exercising like that with my second child. Instead I just did very little movements and stretches and he in turn was more calm."

"Um, thank you for the tip. People are staring, I think we are disrupting the class, better get back into it. Thanks again (nod, nod and smile)."

Going through this profound experience meant doing a lot of 'closet cleaning.' I had to examine my relationship to fear, my relationship to institutional power and authority over my body, my relationship to others (who could I feel very, very safe and exposed around?), as well as my relationship to myself. I would use the time on my yoga blanket each morning to meditate on all of this. A lot of what came up, especially during the first pregnancy, was harsh and raw. Turns out I had a lot of strong feelings, repressed fears and frustration and a lifetime of other emotional debris to clear out. Time after time my pranayama sessions would involve tears of some sort and the resurrecting of old wounds and trespasses from others or even myself that needed forgiving. Luckily no one was around in the early mornings so I was free to be as quiet or expressive as I wanted to be.

I explored my internal world and did a deep dive into my own issues many times during this first pregnancy, somehow feeling the need to purge as much debris as possible before the birth. Looking back, I see that not only was I attempting to bring a healthier version of myself to the birth but to the state of motherhood in general in anticipation of the intense demands it would require. I think I sensed I would no longer have time for long-winding exploratory sessions of self-healing and self-care. If there were major things to explore, any real 'red flags' as it were, I felt the time was 'now.'

Generally speaking, since childhood I had been into health and wellness, but the second I became pregnant I felt deep in my bones that I had to take my health even more seriously. I was inspired to get into the best shape of my life for the sake of the little person growing inside me. I also figured I would feel more confident with muscles I could depend on and an ironclad nervous system. Green spinach or kale smoothies every day and tons of filtered water. Flax seed, plain oatmeal and bean salad hit the menu like never before. Getting plenty of fresh air and sunlight was already a daily affair but now I had an extra excuse to get my behind out of doors more often. I think that despite the risk of taking it all too seriously or having standards set cautiously high, focusing on wellness gave me a lifeline to grip on to as I navigated the seas of uncertainty all around and especially within me. Having no experience as to what a typical healthy pregnancy 'feels' like, it gave me a measure of control and peace of mind to keep doing what made sense and *felt* right.

I stuck like glue to my meditation, breathing and movement framework, never or rarely missing a morning routine, and learned a great deal about myself while sitting in one spot. My wellness routine also included a little each of cardio, postures, stretches and muscle building. This pregnancy situation seemed like a big barrel of undetermined variables, so it was nice to have a nice purchase on my health. I felt like I *could* control avoiding muscle fatigue and lack of stamina, or at least I could certainly try.

I did not start anything totally new, but I certainly did not stop what I was already doing. I was used to listening to what my body needed physically and had long since been into jogging, hiking and going to the gym. I did, however, suddenly become more interested in what my local gym had to offer and talking to fitness buffs about what their pregnancies had been like. I learned to easily modify my movements when I felt the need and to go at my own pace. I attended all sorts of classes, and still enjoyed slow jogging, push-ups, muscle toning and core work. I was at times worried about doing cardio and if that would impact fetal development, but couldn't find much research on the subject. It was easy for me to keep the same pace I always had well into my second trimester. A fitness instructor I knew, who was also a mother, came to my rescue. She found credible studies that showed cardio was safe. I decided to listen to my gut and keep moving my butt. Towards the end of the second trimester I slowed down considerably and just kept doing everything I was doing at a lesser pace.

By the time I gave birth I felt more fit and healthy and had a stronger nervous system than I ever had in my entire life to that point. I had never fully stuck to a daily regime before and the results were incredible. My new found love of squats and chair poses gave me leg strength I had never had before, planks gave me core and upper body strength (which, wow, came in handy during labour as I supported myself on my arms for hours and my muscles never once fatigued), and cardio cleared my mind. My history of back pain was non-existent. My willpower increased along with my muscle mass. That's not to say I didn't have days when I felt crappy and didn't move all that much, but I did try to make sure to move at least a little. I was still totally emotional at times and anxious about the upcoming birth, but taking care of myself gave me a solid outlet for feeling better almost instantly, right until and including the day I gave birth.

Home Birth

To Dance or Not to Dance

Hands down, one of the most transformational events of my life was signing up for a Zumba class during my first pregnancy. It was the only fitness class available that day and I wasn't impressed. I had indigestion, felt crappy and just was not feeling very 'dancy-dancy' in general. I didn't really want to try it. I was positive it wasn't going to challenge me or be much fun at all. The class was always full of smiling people so what the heck, I had nothing to lose. I was in my third month. I stood patiently in the full capacity class, in the back row as usual, trying not to draw attention to my belly, feeling bloated, doubtful, and ready to leave early. But there was hope on the horizon...

In walked Pacco, a tall, dark, charming Mexican man, well-muscled, a smile a mile wide, and one of the most inspiring dancers and group leaders I had ever seen. I had and still have never, ever seen a man shake his thang the way this guy can. He was so happy and supportive and always encouraging us women to move our bodies in a way that was liberating, to have fun, to not take that class (and life!) too seriously, and the list goes on. He used a lot of his own personal favourite tunes over the standard electronic re-made versions and gave intensity options for everyone in the group. He was inclusive, he was having a blast, and was not afraid to laugh at himself or his mistakes. His high-octane energy was intense and addictive, and so was dancing to great music. Suddenly I was back in my living room as an eight-year-old, with the record player blasting, doing cartwheels and headstands and singing out loud having a right jolly old time.

After being introduced to Pacco's class I would find myself in later trimesters, feeling scared or maybe defeated after a long day, downstairs in my rec room dancing along to YouTube videos of *Waka Waka* and *Volare* at full volume. I would dance away for even ten minutes at a time and sweat my butt off, and I even taught some of the routines to my family and nieces just for fun. I was re-awakened to my own passion for movement and music. This fitness teacher, unknowingly, simply by allowing his own passion to shine and by simply doing what he loved to do, was a bright light of empowerment for me. I know that sounds grandiose and over-the-top, but it's the truth. I am forever grateful to Pacco for his gift, which was basically just having the courage to openly be himself, with no pretence, and unapologetically having fun with movement.

Generally I am one to work hard at including everyone and collecting people together. I liked Pacco's butt shaking classes so much I rarely missed one. When it came time to plan my baby shower at the end of my eighth month there was nothing to consider. I had to have Pacco come teach all of us, friends, family, in-laws and work colleagues, some of his great moves! This naturally made my mother have palpitations and the rest of the family raise eyebrows but I didn't care. I knew what would make me happy. And plus, I knew the Pacco magic would rub off. Still hard to believe I now have pictures of our extended families dancing their hearts outside in the sunshine, including those members who had never and would never attend anything close to a fitness class, let alone a dance-themed one. I was struck by the power of movement and music to bring people together, as a universal language and a way to engage everyone.

To be a little cheeky and have some good old-fashioned fun, we followed the dance party with a stroller race amongst the men and then mixed gender (totally hysterical because the plastic baby dolls kept falling out of the strollers, requiring the person to stop and strap them back in properly). We also had wheelbarrow races and a delightful push-up contest (I did not partake), children's games and tons of great food.

I followed Pacco during my second and third pregnancies as well. By the third pregnancy, he would introduce me to the whole dance class, playfully pointing out my pregnant belly (usually I was the only obviously pregnant dancer) and even telling the participants to follow me instead of him. When it was time for my third baby shower we went big and bold one more time and Pacco taught us to dance again. This time around I was a tad bit more pregnant than the first shower. I had just started my ninth month. My good friend and her husband designed cool co-gender signs and decorations. By now I had many more friends with babies and toddlers all over the place and there were plenty of children dancing along with us. Though I promised to modify what I was doing so that I could enjoy myself without overdoing it, my mother made me smile by hiding in the kitchen and telling everyone, "Oh my God, I can't even watch this. I am just going to hide here doing the dishes!" It was a big memorable party, and I still can't think of it without feeling emotional. I was touched when my eldest sister warmly described the meaning of our celebration in her own words, saying that I was 'dancing my child into the world.'

Meditation and Other Complications

"Hey, by the way, did you know that she's pregnant?"

"Seriously?"

"Um, yeah."

"But she's not married yet!"

"Seriously Jeremy? It's 2012."

Silence

"And anyways, neither are you!"

"But I don't have any kids yet!"

I find it inspiring to learn as much about health and wellness as possible, to feel the relief, power and potential that come with learning about the choices and options that are out there. By the time I had become pregnant I had been practicing yoga and meditation for at least 7 years. By practicing I mean not only going to a class each week (which I did), I mean trying my best to integrate the classical yogic principles and philosophy into my life. I'm a pretty logical gal and everything about yoga, as it was presented to me, just simply made sense. It felt as though I already knew, on some level, everything that I was learning from my teachers, as though I was simply re-learning it all. I talk about this in my journey here because it really was a key pillar in all three of my home birth journeys.

As fate would have it, I found myself in a kundalini yoga class when I started to take my yoga and wellness practice outside of my home. A kundalini class is not like most typical yoga classes in North America, it's nothing like anything I had seen before, anywhere. It is called the fitness of the future as it combines movement, breathing and meditation all at once for maximum efficiency. A lot of the exercises are done seated, with eyes closed or almost closed most of the time. The energy of the room has a mindful, almost sacred tone, as people are encouraged to go deep within and clean out their cobwebs, so to speak. Our beautiful teacher Anina created a space, a time container, which allowed us to feel comfortable really digging deep sometimes, being usual or unusual, or whatever we needed to be on a particular day. She is a brave and powerful leader and at the time I didn't realize just how much courage and vulnerability it can take to create and foster an environment like this.

I dove right in excitedly, wide open to what I might learn. I was sitting in my first class off to the side, towards the back, the lighting very dim. All was quiet. Everyone including the teacher had their eyes closed, then we were asked to perform breath of fire, a very rapid breath done through the nose. I could hear the guy beside me breathing very loudly, almost making a snorting sound. Um, what did I get myself into?

Soon the teacher said, "Okay, now we will simply sit and mediate for five full minutes in silence." Say what? You mean sit still doing absolutely nothing with our eyes closed for *5 full minutes*? Like no moving or making a sound? How about some music please? I did it, it was worth it, and I realized then and there that if this was a challenge, simply sitting in silence, it was likely what I needed to work on most. To learn to be still. To re-learn to breathe properly and in a multitude of ways. I was challenged, frustrated, and completely sold. I went to every single one of my teacher's classes. Each Tuesday evening became the time I had my weekly energy vitamins. I couldn't explain at that point why the class worked to energize and calm and seemingly heal me, but I definitely felt better every time I attended. This style of yoga would become a component of my regular health and teaching regime. I would also use the exercises as a way to warm up before sports or dancing and I began to practice meditation at home. I loved the way the specific movements 'unlocked' my back and made my spine instantly less stiff.

As mainstream as western yoga is, I was surprised how much the rest of the ancient practices and explicit pranayama (breathing techniques) are not. This has been made painfully obvious to me more than once. Of all the habits I have felt the need to visually hide from others in my life, I am continually surprised that meditation is one of them. I am not sure what is so weird about it, yet I've grown used to it drawing attention and some of the scenarios I've found myself in are quite comical.

Not that long ago I found a very private shaded spot along a lovely little river to sit and go through my pranayama exercises. A lovely family with four small children happened upon me. The mother smiled lovingly at me, babe in arms, while her husband taught the children about the foliage around us. All was serene at first as I continued doing my own thing, but when I began performing kapalabhati (a more forceful breathing technique that focuses on the exhale), you would have thought I had sprouted two heads. I opened my eyes to the same woman looking horrified and confused as she quickly started shuffling her children away from me. It was just like the scene in *Frozen* where Olaf thinks Kristoff has lost his mind for talking to rocks (that turn out to be trolls) and calmly tries to get Anna to walk away as fast as possible. It was both funny, sad and ironic at the same time.

I found myself on another occasion searching for anywhere to sit outdoors where I could have a little privacy. I was at a friend's house in a very small town and the yard was tiny. I found the most secluded spot I could to the right of the house and driveway, my view from the street mostly blocked by a parked car. I sat in stillness and started to do my own thing, becoming nice and relaxed. Holy crap, out of nowhere something hairy climbed on top of me and I shrieked my brains out. It was a very friendly neighbourhood cat. Okay. Breathe. It's all good.

I started to gradually relax again. Not five minutes later I was startled by footsteps and a deep voice. The neighbour to the left came running across his lawn, looking concerned. Was I okay? Why were my eyes closed? Did I need medical support? Was I sure? Was I *really* sure? Honestly, what was I supposed to say to him? *"No, actually I was deeply relaxed until you popped my bubble."* I thanked him and, feeling embarrassed, decided to walk to the local café for a cup of tea. Sure enough, that same man who had just come to see if I was okay was the person who served me at the counter. This was getting funny now. And naturally, he made sure to ask once again if I was 'okay,' just in case. Speechless. Eyes downcast. *Just keep swimming. Just keep swimming.*

It's interesting to reflect on the parts of my personality that interplay in these types of situations; mainstream norms and my desire for peace and acceptance battle with my thirst for sharing knowledge and normalizing traditional health practices. These different components seem to constantly compete, regroup, compete again, and often, if I am honest, the safety of silence wins out. My not wanting to draw attention to myself for doing something different collides with an urging to go ahead and do it anyways regardless of what others may think. For a long time I have had mixed emotions about rocking the mainstream proverbial boat. Whether we are talking about meditation, or natural medicine, or ancient technology, or being fully informed, I seem to walk a thin line between two worldviews, creating a bit of a hybrid that places me in neither world completely. I have wondered if other people, especially women and mothers, feel this way too, or is my own unique sensitivity to blame?

Yoga, the Old School Way

About two years after starting my kundalini practice fate dumped me at the doorstep of my next teacher. Of course I had no idea at the time that's what was happening. Well apparently I was ready for the next level on all levels because my new teacher, whom I simply called Guru Dev, was a no-nonsense, no time-wasting, blunt, direct, loving, firm, teacher of the old ways. He himself had been studying and practicing for many decades. A distinguished Indian gentleman new to Canada, he introduced me to a classical view and traditional concept of yoga. It was an instant connection at first site for me. He had not taken on an 'official' dedicated student before in Canada (and boy did he insist that I and his future students be dedicated). I was interested and open to learning what yoga was about really, historically, and as a technology for health. His teachings had a major impact on my life choices, lifestyle and routine. The time slot he offered me for our weekly yoga sessions was 5:15 am. Okay then. Groan. I am not going to lie. This was not an easy adjustment for a night owl like myself to say the least. Dragging my butt out of bed that early and then hitting the daily grind with a full workday afterwards was totally challenging and demanded a lot of discipline. He would be up and ready to greet me at the door looking as though he had been awake for hours (well he had been, he usually began his morning yoga at 3:30 am).

At first I was only allowed to take all the information in by listening to him speak for hours and couldn't write anything down. I learned about vibration, mantra, pranayama (breathing techniques), philosophy, movement, meditation, how to live yoga and apply it to daily life, creating a less harmful lifestyle, nutrition and food preparation and tons more (books full actually). A lot of what I learned felt like I was re-learning what I already knew. I was taught that consistently working with the breath in a disciplined way could, theoretically, assist with healing, preventing and potentially cure many physical, emotional and mental ailments. But I had to put things into practice; my teacher often said yoga is 99% discipline and effort and 1% grace. The results were great. I cannot remember ever even coming down with a serious cold while doing the breathing exercises regularly.

I learned the main focus of yoga as it was intended is not on performing postures or physical flexibility but rather befriending the mind. We did some posture work and physical movement, but my teacher's focus was really on claiming power over our minds and yogic philosophy. He told me I could go anywhere at all to learn about postures and didn't want to therefore waste my time when he knew I wouldn't find his teachings elsewhere. Progress was very gradual. We started simply learning about Aum, the primordial healing vibration. Then how to use it while breathing as a mantra. Then we learned about long deep breathing, kapalabhati, and analoom-valoom (alternate nostril breathing), the three primary breaths to be used every single day, and then other multiple breaths that would be put together into a set each day. A daily at-home routine slowly developed that, if done as prescribed, easily took over an hour.

Gradually a few other male students joined us, and by the time I was in my first pregnancy I had been doing the practice for a few years. The class timing had (luckily) shifted to the weekends and much later in the morning. That was my weekly pre-natal yoga! Sitting with three other men, all of us dressed in white, learning about philosophy and taking notes for hours, practicing breathing techniques and meditating together and sipping ghee mixed with honey and pressed organic ginger. It was lovely. I always left feeling better and reminded of what was most important in life.

I was mostly able to continue the prescribed practice (with necessary modifications like avoiding stomach pumping), right up until the day I gave birth. Though I often found it challenging to continue to get up early and do this every single day, the habit of doing so did wondrous things for my health and outlook on life. It also seriously helped me with pre-natal anxiety and worries, of which I had many. I really felt I had been given a secret key to wellness. Of course, at this point I had no idea just how lucky I was to have the child-free time for doing all this wellness work.

I trained with Guru Dev weekly for about five years and then sporadically for a few more until he basically set me free, saying I was ready to become a teacher myself, even though at the time that idea seemed somehow out of reach to me. He gave of his time and space completely, freely and with dedication, all for free. Even when we insisted on bringing him some kind of gift to reciprocate the generosity, he would suggest we bring him a flower. He remains a treasured guide and I am deeply grateful for all the wisdom, patience and guidance he shared over the years.

And here is a little side note about my yoga teacher:

Born in a much warmer climate than found here in Canada, he faced an entirely different life than I did. He is multilingual and well-educated and especially well-versed in the philosophical context of yoga. And he puts it into practice (as in up at 3:00 am for a few hours or practice before making breakfast and then repeat again for a few more hours in the evening). Once, I asked him a direct parenting question. (This was at a time when I was uncertain on my parenting feet, trying to deal with judgment and criticism from internal and external sources and a million different voices that seemed to be telling me that maybe I shouldn't follow my gut). The question was about co-sleeping and should the baby *actually* be sleeping alone through the night by now? I was agonizing over getting rid of the dammed crib that my daughter refused to sleep in. I was comfortable with her next to me, which was the only place she wanted to be anyways. I'm sleep-deprived and nursing every 45 minutes and somehow I still found the time to care that "everyone will judge me, won't they?" Sadly, I hadn't yet found the amazing tribe of attachment parents I now run with, who share similar values and all support one another. I was feeling a complete lack of support and was trying to make the best possible choices. I knew what my gut was saying was right but still sought approval from others. So I asked my teacher: "How old were you when your mother put you in a separate room to sleep at night?"

He looked at me directly and paused with a half-smile and I will never forget his words or how they humbled me. "My dear Cera. My mother was 14 when she had me and I was the first of 7 children. We lived in a one room house, like most people in our village, and I lived there my whole young life until I was old enough to move out for school." Case closed.

And here is another sidebar: As I explained earlier, when I started learning with this teacher everything was very, very old school. I basically had to sit and mentally take in tons of information, like they did in the old days. It was the way he himself had been taught for years. If I got too cramped up or tired we would do a little bit of movement or stretches and then straight back to learning, studying the texts, memorizing verses and prayers and poems, working with our breath and learning recipes. Later on we had to write everything out by hand in duplicate into a special book of records that we looked after with extreme care. We didn't interrupt and we didn't disagree. We were humble and learning to discipline ourselves.

Later on, after taking an extended break from the class to have a baby, I returned to join an expanded group and lo and behold! Class was now half the length of time to accommodate everyone's busy schedules! People were being given handouts!!, *including extra copies if they misplaced anything*. One person even typed up everything my teacher taught on a *laptop!* Then they got to move (!) for the second half of the class while he led them in stretches and postures. Someone had to leave a little early or come a little late? *No problem.*

I feel the way I was made to study helped carve me into the person I am today. I do sometimes have mixed emotions looking back on everything, realizing I had found a teacher whose drive and approach matched my own stratospheric expectations that I had placed on myself. For instance, I felt disappointed and disillusioned when I could no longer 'keep up,' I felt disappointed and even a little bit disillusioned. Never wanting to throw the baby out with the bathwater meant I would, over time, lighten up, learn not to put anyone on a holy pedestal, take the good I learned for all it was worth, and be able to smile at the whole adventure, such that it was. An adventure in discipline, inner exploration and a whole new way of experiencing life.

Home Birth

Finding New Standards

With the arrival of a baby, suddenly my commitment to my own health and wellness took a major back seat. It was more important to support her and be emotionally available than to focus on myself each morning. Was I the weird one for thinking I couldn't meet the previous standards I has unknowingly set for myself? It made me think of my grandmother and her mother before her. Pioneer women in this country. No indoor bathrooms, winter in northern Ontario, eight months pregnant, and having to go out at night to feed the animals in the barn their supper after feeding three kids in the house. Might I add my grandmother had to climb up and down a staircase in the unheated barn, in the dark, while holding large mounds of hay!? Preposterous.

My second pregnancy saw me doing different activities than the first. For starters, being pregnant in the winter is way different than in summer where I live. Furthermore, I now had a very independent toddler who simply would no longer go into a stroller or a carrier for more than five minutes. Finding time for self-care was certainly more challenging now. Whereas outdoor walks during my third trimester had been my solace in my first pregnancy, I found myself deeply annoyed and frustrated by both the weather and the lack of cooperation from my toddler. Eventually I had to get creative. My body was craving the outlet of long leisurely walks and it finally hit me! Home renovation stores! I'm not kidding. Whenever we had or even didn't have any ad-hoc shopping to do in these huge stores, I would happily park my daughter in the cart and stroll up and down the isles for twenty minutes just to let my legs move! Then I would go outside if it wasn't snowing and do the same thing in the parking lot. If anyone else thought it was funny that an 8-month pregnant woman was pushing an empty shopping cart with a toddler in it around and around and around a parking lot, in the dark, they never said anything.

I continued my morning yoga although the timeframe was often reduced substantially. I would squeeze in small meditation bursts whenever I could, including going into the stairwell at work at lunch or sometimes sitting on the floor behind my desk. I enjoyed and was able to maintain this practice almost every single day right up until the birth of my second child and then 'poof,' I just couldn't meet the standards anymore. Too busy with the caring for two babies full time, too much else to focus on, I really hadn't realized just how much pressure I had put on myself. For a long time I felt disappointed in myself as I was still mentally holding myself to my teacher's high standards, for what I perceived as falling short. There was no exception for motherhood in the regime I was following. You simply found a way to keep to your schedule. It needed to be the most important thing. Gradually, though it would take a while, I realized that whatever I could do, no matter how small or large, was good enough, especially when parenting small children. I now just try to do whatever I can, no matter how little time I have. I can now say that I have lightened up more and learned to have creative fun with this yoga business.

During my third pregnancy I continued to practice the pranayama and meditation exercises whenever I could, but certainly not every day, and by that point I was almost totally okay with that. By then I also had a regular teaching practice which was expanding. I was delighted to be asked to teach pre-natal yoga for expecting women while I was pregnant myself.

If I could go back to that time now I would be much more accepting of where I was in my life. I would actually stop and take the time to congratulate myself for the things I had accomplished and not focus on what I was unable to do. Like motherhood for instance, especially rooted in the attachment parenting philosophy. Eventually taking care of my kids became my new way of practicing yoga, of being of service.

I think of my own mother, a teacher and school principal, who took years off the job to give birth to and raise five children, and the realities she faced. She was in university when pregnant with me and then used to go home from her teaching job during her lunch hour to nurse me in the months after I was born. I used to have so much more judgment of my parents, 'why weren't they more this and that and the other,' mostly because I did not have the experience to know better.

Having kids is, well, kind of insane sometimes, and most of all demanding. I would not have described myself as a feminist before, and I very much support the mothering cause now. Maybe I would call myself a 'familyist.' As a mother, I felt it was necessary, yet as a professional I felt guilty and awkward for leaving work early to take time to get physically and mentally ready for delivering a baby. I tried to explain this concept to management but just couldn't articulate my reasons very well. It was as though the language to do so didn't exist.

It was very difficult to try to explain what I needed and why, believe it or not. I was challenged and would need to provide documentation. I was compared to other women who 'worked until the day they gave birth.' I had no doubt I probably could have, theoretically, but to what end? What was I trying to prove by doing that? The short-term investment of time off to stay healthy and strong before labour for long-term gain made natural sense to me but not logical sense to some others in our capitalist society. Every step of the family making and rearing process is a major accomplishment in my view, one that is greatly undervalued. My hat is off in the grandest salute to all parents who gave and continue to give everything they possibly can to their families.

Home Birth

Keeping Things Secret Sometimes

"Knock, knock." I pause what I was doing to look up at a new, lovely, direct and not so subtle friend of mine. I am caught off guard somehow, knowing this is not going to be a usual conversation in any way. "I just wanted to let you know why I don't seem to be happy and I won't be congratulating you on your pregnancy."

Um, okay. Very awkward silence on my end. How did she know? I have barely told anyone! Did she guess? Man word gets around fast over here!

She continued without hesitating: "When something that you want so badly to happen doesn't no matter how hard you try, it's just really hard to be around someone else who has what you want." More awkward silence before I find my voice. Diffusing the awkward tension is my first goal. "Thank you for telling me, I respect how you must feel." We chat awhile longer about her serious long-term struggle. The prognosis was bleak. I'm feeling partly frustrated that others around me cannot share in my happiness, but I am also seeing a bigger picture of possibilities. Maybe we were together to learn from each other. Who knows, maybe my pregnancy pheromones would even have a positive role here. I mentally send her all the encouragement and hope that I can. I try my best to believe in her dream. We gradually, day-by-day, become closer and closer and my pregnancy seems to become a non-issue after all. So different yet so similar we are.

I couldn't have been happier, really, when a year and a half later I bump into her and lo and behold, she has a delightful babe in arms. I am shocked and delighted and deeply inspired. They had surmounted tremendous odds. Life found a way.

At first we kept things to ourselves, yes, but gradually as the safety time zone of the first trimester passed I was proud and happy to be visibly pregnant almost anywhere. With a few exceptions. Not everyone was open to the idea of an at-home birth. Further, there is a subtle aspect to being a pregnant person that is lesser acknowledged. During my graduate courses one of my classmates discussed her topic of women being pregnant in public. How they often felt they received the message that, well, maybe they shouldn't 'be' in public. I was intrigued by her work and the resulting discussion in the classroom. I really had never examined my own view and perspectives on pregnant women up to that point. I certainly noticed them, especially when they were in late pregnancy. It made me examine more of the dogma that exists within me and us all, the remnants of previous centuries of judgments about what is suitable and what is not for women. Overall, being very sympathetic to the feminist cause, I felt that women should do what they like, as equals to others, pregnant or not.

And so I did. Most of the time people were respectful. As my belly grew bigger I did sometimes feel like something of a novelty. If you want to get some attention fast, simply assume plank pose or push-up position in a room with other people in it when you are more than eight months pregnant. The reactions can range from complete fear to downright hysterical. Overall I sensed a mixture of curiosity, surprise, encouragement, and judgmental energy when I was out in public and very visibly pregnant. It often changed depending on what I was doing. I was usually the only visibly pregnant woman still sweating my butt off and having fun during the fitness classes. Because I genuinely was having fun I suppose I drew even more attention.

Here and there I noticed a few sideways glances that weren't always very encouraging. The one and only kickboxing aerobics class I took was when I was four months pregnant. It was the only thing they were offering that day and I needed to move. I thought about not going but decided I may as well try it out. My female partner absolutely refused to continue partnering with me once she noticed I was pregnant. I didn't know what to do and just did drills on my own. Another time I was doing squats with a small medicine ball when a trainer surprised me by scooping it right out of my hands and replaced it with a smaller softer one, without saying anything to me. Awkward, awkward. Awkward.

I remember one day another class member actually interrupted me during a popular fitness class while I was dancing and feeling great. On this particular day I was doing the same thing I usually did when I exercised, which was almost the exact same thing as everyone else just in a modified, lower-impact style. No jumping or anything that bothered my belly in the least. I had gotten good at figuring out ways to make myself sweat through engaging my muscles deeply without shaking my whole body around. Another woman took my arm gently and pulled me to the side of the group mid-song. I gave her my full attention assuming it must be urgent. She then told me I should reconsider my moves and lower my intensity, since she had done the same when she was pregnant and her baby then turned out to be overly 'alert' and moved a lot more than her other children, and someone had told her it was likely because of the way she had exercised. Stunned, I noticed people were starting to stare, and not wanting to argue the point in such a public situation, I thanked her, smiled, and got on with the class. But my shiny happy enthusiastic mood was now gone.

After this incident I became increasingly self-conscious. The subtle message I often received once I was really showing a bump was that I should be walking and stretching for the most part. Sometimes I felt like maybe I shouldn't be in the gym at all. I already was someone who liked to stick to the back row and do my own thing, and now I felt even more so this way. I tried to literally shrink my energy field so that I wouldn't be noticed as much, wore darker colours and tried to make it look like I wasn't working as hard as I was. I learned to avoid 'letting it rip,' primarily in case I made someone else around me uncomfortable.

People seemed to 'notice' an obviously pregnant woman working out in a traditionally masculine way. I remember eventually going into the fire escape stairwell during my lunch hour to do some exercise in privacy. It wasn't used that much and I figured I would have the privacy I craved. I had had enough of the scrutiny. Plank and push-ups were what always seemed to make people nervous the most. It was almost comical.

One, two, three, almost done number four, then *creek, whoosh,* I hear the door opening. I scramble to get up off the floor but it is too late! The co-worker who usually sat beside me walked in mid-sentence with some colleagues. I gulped and turned beet-red. *Busted! Caught in the act doing push-ups with nowhere to hide.* Why was I wondering if he was going to tell on me! In the end he had the graciousness not to say anything. I could, however, see a twinkle in his eyes.

I started to seek out any other private corners that I could find to move, stretch, or get the blood moving. I really felt the need to move and to do so often, and I just didn't want to feel noticed anymore.

There is also a certain sense of vulnerability that comes with being visibly pregnant. When I was really, really pregnant for the first time it was late summer. It was very hot and very dry outside. I walked every day for sunlight, fresh air, and to relax. One time a group of young men made some loud unwanted comments as I walked by which embarrassed and intimidated me.

I was passing a new house construction site wearing a tank top several days before my due date. One young man came extremely close to my face to 'congratulate' me loudly in front of the others. I sensed this was coming as he approached me, despite trying to mind my own business and not start a conversation in any way.

Then there was a more serious incident that happened during my second pregnancy, when I was just starting to show. I wanted to get some fresh air and exercise during a stressful day at work. I passed a man sitting on a park bench in a forested area who set off my danger instincts as he too closely watched me pass by. I chose to get the exercise I wanted, my annoyance with being restricted outweighing my urge for caution. I decided not to put fear above my need to be where I was and ignored warning bells going off inside. I went off the path a little to a spot I felt offered a little privacy. Sure enough once I started my short workout I could see him through the trees coming towards me. Looked like he was smiling in a weird sort of way. I felt more unnerved than scared, not able to get a solid reading from what exactly he wanted or intended. He moved a little closer, and I felt temporarily frozen as I was forced to evaluate my safety options and decided that my speed would likely be my only weapon in the circumstance.

It was November and no one else was around *except,* out of nowhere, a cyclist all in black appeared on the path, stopped suddenly, and called immediately for me to join him. I didn't hesitate moving closer to him and I could sense his energy was unusually protective and alert somehow, purposeful perhaps. He insisted I walk back to the parking lot area with him, explaining along the way that he was an undercover police officer ensuring safety in the area which had seen some recent crimes against female path-users. He told me not to go out and exercise alone like that again. He said he had been looking for and recognized the person who had been trying to approach me (who took off pretty quickly at that point). I was quite shaken after this event, extremely grateful yet also indignant and angry. Angry at myself for putting myself in that situation. Had I 'attracted' the danger? Wasn't it stupid to see warning bells and go walking forward anyways? How dare someone chase me. Mostly I was pissed off about the double standard in society and general lack of safety women sometimes experience in these types of areas. I could not seemingly go out for some exercise when I wanted, on my own terms, without being constantly attuned to the possibility of danger. Like being punished for trying to do something healthy for yourself.

Unfortunately over time a second similar situation occurred. Collectively these incidents forced me to re-evaluate the way I would approach exercise and enjoy nature. My teacher used to say that a single fly can contaminate an entire pail of milk. During my whole life nature had been nothing but a refuge, if anything the one place I usually *was feeling* totally safe. I used to spend hours alone in the woods at Grandma's or behind our home, picking berries and playing and not giving it a second thought. Everything was turned on its head in a matter of minutes. I know some folks might shake their heads at this kind of talk and maybe pass it off as being in denial or being privileged, entitled or naïve. *Obviously* there is danger on a bike path in November. Normal. Or is it? Is it *obviously* something we women should *have* to be on the lookout for constantly? Or is it so much a normal part of our functioning, especially once we become parents, that we don't notice our own hypervigilance anymore?

Another awkward experience came while

having breakfast at a golf club. A much older man who appeared to be somewhat into his cups was staring at me pointedly and eventually loudly barked across the patio from his table: *"Yer about 7 months aren't ya? I'm the king of measuring pregnant bellies, ah ha ha."* I am still at a loss for words all these years later.

And then there is applying for a new job when you are already pregnant, right at that perfect time when you are just beginning to show and it is still usually rude to ask a woman about it because there is a good chance you could be wrong.

My work unit had been disbanded and we were all tasked with finding new jobs as soon as possible. I had a really caring, protective and supportive manager behind me and I am eternally grateful. One day he mentioned offhandedly, "It's not like you are pregnant again and will need to leave the new job right after you start." Moral dilemma. Does he know or does he already suspect? Should I come clean? I decided to tell him privately and was glad for it, because I think he put extra energy towards helping me get quickly established elsewhere by means of reference.

Hiring discrimination against pregnant women is not allowed. However that didn't mean it doesn't happen. One good friend of mine pulled me aside one day. I hadn't told her I was pregnant but I instantly knew she just knew. She quietly told me she had recently been offered a position in writing, and when she let them know of her pregnancy suddenly the position was re-titled and they no longer had the funding to hire her. She told me to "keep my books in front of my belly" when I went for interviews.

I wasn't overly stressed about finding a new job, at first that is. I was still doing my breathing practices every morning and taking things well in stride overall. Then it came time for interviews and a few great offers came in. I knew my legal rights, I didn't need to disclose anything, but still I also felt keeping something so obvious to myself was misleading, as in: *"Hi! You just hired me and I am so grateful. Please note I will do my very best to be a great team member for the full three months I plan to be here!"* I really did want to start off on a very honest footing with my new work team.

My final interview was with a prestigious organization. It had always seemed out of reach to me somehow but I applied anyways figuring I had nothing to lose. The level of competition to join their team was fierce and I knew many people who wanted to work there. You needed to be bilingual and have a Master's degree at minimum to apply, yet almost all of the people I knew working there had one or two PhD's and many were multi-lingual. During the interview I sat at a table surrounded by eight lovely people. The whole management team it seemed came out to meet and interview me. My quasi-bump was just barely camouflaged by the table I sat at. I had a dark green shirt on. Should I pretend to stretch and stand up and make it obvious? Should I say nothing and hope for the best? In the end I decided to neither hide it nor announce it. I was totally stressed to the point that I may actually have appeared very relaxed and nonchalant (I really thought I wasn't going to get this job).

Funny how when we feel we are completely out of our league we sometimes rise to the occasion. I must have won them over. I just really wanted to walk into a brand new position without any unnecessary guilt or tension. The next day I received a phone call from the manager. She offered me the job. I was delighted and accepted. I was feeling nervous and totally chicken but I took a breath and told her the truth about my pregnant state of affairs, and when I would need to be leaving on maternity. Because I felt so guilty at the time I also promised I would harbour no ill will and take no action if she decided not to hire me after all. I really gave her every possible opening to back out of the deal!

Then there was a *very* long pause.

Oh man. I literally bit down on my inside lower lip to avoid speaking and started mentally counting to ten. There was a very audible deep breath on the other end of the line, then: "Okay, well I will think it over and get back to you." Yeah, not the best sleep of my life that evening I can tell you.

The following day I was invited to a meeting where the female Executive was present. I could almost immediately sense that there was a different climate, a different type of energy here compared to the work environments I was used to, though I couldn't put my finger on it exactly. I had no clue what to expect and sat with baited breath; were they still going to hire me? The suspense was brutal. The meeting began and the voice of the female Executive rang out confidently and true, firm, in charge, and to the point:

"First of all congratulations are in order, Cera, we hear you are expecting. Secondly, welcome to the team. Please know that we would never consider changing our mind about your offer, a woman's work value or ability to be hired should never be based on whether or not she's having a baby. Moving on!"

My jaw dropped, I was a little blown away, and inwardly delighted. The hiring manager looked slightly uncomfortable but said nothing. Is this how a female ship gets run? A sense that I would be okay on this team crept in. And I was, and they were, and I rejoiced to have joined a group of very hardworking, passionate and caring people. I still felt entirely out of my league of course but I learned what I could, as fast as I could, and did the best that I could during the time I was there.

Fear All Around Us

I am working silently on a document. The walls are paper thin around here. This would be one of those times when I wondered why I was put where I was when I was. This would be a time when I was afraid of not minding my own business. A beautiful colleague of mine is pregnant and I hear her chatting on the phone. It sounds serious. My ears prick up. It gets quiet for a moment, then I can hear her quietly sobbing. Oh no. My skin prickles, my heart rate speeds up, please don't let this be something serious with her baby. Her voice cracks as she leaves a tearful voice mail for her husband asking him to please call her back right away.

Something is very wrong. Should I or shouldn't I? I know her well but not 'well' well. Will I be crossing the line? Or will it be worse if I pretend I heard nothing? I just can't leave her to face whatever it is totally alone. I take the chance and nervously approach her door and hesitate, ready to leave in haste if that is what she prefers. She welcomes my company at her side but keeps crying into her hands. I feel helpless. I send all the positive energy I possibly can towards her and the baby. Eventually she tells me that someone just told her her unborn baby most likely has a serious and potentially fatal heart defect.

Over the next few days and weeks I see her muster up some determined, positive energy. She tells me they asked for a second opinion from a specialist they know who works in a prestigious institute. In the end it was a false alarm.

Looking back from my current vantage point I see all the aspects about birth, pregnancy, child-rearing and other women-centred roles from a totally new perspective. Or maybe it is more accurate to say my eyes are now open. It may go without saying that the first pregnancy and birth I experienced presented me with unknowns every day. The fear of the great unknown and the deeply instilled, and even subconscious fear of childbirth was the biggest obstacle I faced. Adjusting my mindset, my beliefs and ways of thinking was the largest part of the pregnancy work. Really. Suddenly fear slapped me upside the face from every direction possible. Exacerbating this was my challenge in finding positive role models who were courageous and happy instead of simply cautious.

Every health appointment during pregnancy, from acupressure, physio and even all the midwife appointments, included a discussion and overview of risks and worse case scenarios. Everyone wants a pregnant woman to be cautious and I naturally agree with this. Growing a life is a privilege, a tremendous responsibility and is generally awe-inspiring and I certainly took it seriously. However, it did not make sense to go around being anxious or worried about doing the right or wrong thing all the time. Also I wondered, if pregnancy was a completely natural event we are designed for, why was it treated as a medical condition? Most medical conditions are unwanted, aren't they?

Growing up I thought about birth and tried to make sense of what it was all really about. I heard the typical horror stories about birth, whether the focus was the lack of privacy or empathy from nameless staff in birthing rooms or actual physical trauma, and it all had the same effect on me. This stuff sounded scary. Period. Even if I had heard positive stories or even neutral ones, which I am sure I occasionally did, my memories would just default to the many scary ones, until very recently that is.

Then there was all the media and movies over the years that had left a tragic imprint in my mind. I think it was at a family drive-in where I saw Spock being born during the *Star Trek* movie (what not to watch while you are pregnant). And whether it was *Star Trek* or *Star Wars* or comedies or simple TV episodes, the common narrative seemed to include a screaming, distressed, often irrational woman, on her back, overwhelming people around her as she angrily battled labour pains and endured a serious lack of personal privacy, the latter many times being portrayed as 'hilarious.' Suffering greatly just sounded like a price we had to pay to become a parent, or something women just had to accept as was their due. Did I really have to go through this to produce a child? I really didn't like the idea of having my power taken away from me or being scarred forevermore on some level.

Many verbal anecdotes that came my way seemed to be centred around pain, fear, lack of respect, a lack of support or empathy or the loss of autonomy and decision making power. I recently accompanied a very close friend during the birth of her second child and unfortunately saw some of these things firsthand, including a lack of empathy and sensitivity to my friend's emotional and physical needs that was startling. My friend seemingly needed permission to do simple things like change position and really wasn't consulted with all that much. Strangers showed up during the birth then would leave again, without introduction, explanation or eye contact, despite the acutely personal situation that was going on, my friend's partial nudity and her desire for privacy. I wanted to somehow protect her privacy and dignity but felt it wasn't my place to argue with philosophical practices that were heavily entrenched.

All of this helped foster a complete and total unconscious fear of birth that would take years and much effort to heal.

As I mentioned, my own mother had gone through some physical and emotional trauma as had my grandmother, and my aunt's and sibling's birth stories weren't much more inspiring. Nearly every birth story involved some close call with trauma or death. These horror stories unfortunately got passed down through my genes and oral history. Thank goodness my grandmother and my mother somehow found their strength and courage to do it again and produced four more healthy babies or I wouldn't be here telling this story. In the case of my mother, starting with baby number three she started getting the hang of things and asserting herself. She started refusing medication and when staff asked her to hold back and not push my older brother into the world until they could run and get the doctor she ignored them and let her body take the lead. By the time I rolled around, baby number 4, she had transformed fully! She also, I am told, had a loving, patient doctor. She knew by now she could take charge, refuse interventions (she did) and could take her own time. Because of experience she was not scared anymore and also my dad was allowed in the room by then. My birth was quick and easy, apparently I was very quiet upon arrival, no fanfare, and I just sort of smiled while turning my head towards the sound of my mother's voice. No one insisted I 'cry' and so I didn't. What can I say?

Changing the Channel

"Seriously this feels like such a hopeless situation long-term. I am so worried now. I am starting to freak out!!"

(Soft tone) "Cera, trust your knowing!"

My long-term Physiotherapist and Osteopath specializes in reproductive issues. I went to see her years before becoming pregnant, after being diagnosed with a potential blockage in my fallopian tube. I was told at the time the only option was exploratory surgery and to keep monitoring. After receiving this horrible news I remember sitting outside the clinic and experiencing a moment of sheer panic, thinking all kinds of worst case scenarios for my childbearing future. I felt like I couldn't breathe properly and faced a dead end. Yet this route just didn't make sense. There had to be a different way somehow, despite my fear that maybe there just wasn't. Suddenly I had a strong sense of knowing come over me that made me pause and turn inwards. Despite my panic my intuition was making noise and urging me to investigate further. And I did. I Googled, I asked questions, I read. The answer would come through the gentle hands of a healer and via a process I knew very little to nothing about.

As fate would have it, I was seeing an Osteopath at the time. She unfortunately didn't have experience with pelvic floor or specific reproductive issues and so she passed me along to my current practitioner who is both a qualified osteopath and physiotherapist with many years of experience in both private and hospital settings. Getting an appointment might have been luck or my desperation for good help shining through because I was told in no uncertain terms this practitioner was too busy to take any new clients. The woman who was treating me kindly called in person and explained my situation to her specialist colleague who agreed to start seeing me as she felt that she could likely help me. Somehow one appointment led to many, many more. To my joy and surprise within a few short months of hands-on physio my swollen, distended, potentially partially blocked fallopian tube was almost completely back to its normal condition. The light but constant ache, the fluid build-up and swelling, gone. Interestingly, so was my fear. Perhaps this was due to the confidence that comes with working with a practitioner who has already helped people in this situation in the past. Although an ultrasound still showed some distention or stretching, the organ once again 'felt' normal I was told and likely wouldn't cause me any difficulty. What technology could show via an ultrasound picture my physiotherapist could 'feel' and very gently manipulate with her hands. I began to more fully understand just how the body is always trying to heal itself, and that removing physical tension and stress around and within an organ, muscle or other body part supports the body in restoring a state of balance.

My physiotherapist/osteopath would see me each month during my pregnancies, do gentle adjustments as needed and would help ensure that things were on track. I enjoyed my relaxing sessions and felt reassured after each session with her. Through her ministrations she helped my body and brain to be ready for birth. She treated me right until the tail end of pregnancy. (She also did craniosacral work on my children after birth, along with any follow-up osteo/physio after birth treatment that I needed). While she was supportive and non-judgmental, she was clear at one point that she didn't think 'Home' was in any way a safe environment for birth. She had a very different and valid perspective to share and she felt the risk was too great. I completely respected her opinion. And she respected mine, all three times I chose to deliver at home. She continues to be a treasured support to me and my family.

I was determined there could be a better way forward than entertaining my and everyone else's fear *all the time*. I didn't want to be scared anymore.

I didn't want to believe pregnancy was a medical problem a doctor had to attend to. I didn't want to believe that my body needed intervention because it didn't know what to do. I wanted some new beliefs!

I continued to turn my attention to the more optimistic stories, feeling that my viewpoint and focus would have a large role on the outcome I wanted to see. I sometimes see fear as helpful and other times like a virus that spreads and warps the truth. There's a beautiful saying by Henry Ford that I like to lean on sometimes: *"Whether you think you can, or whether you think you can't, either way you are right."*

I needed to consciously turn away from fear-based stories, messages and media. There were extremely popular pregnancy books I now avoided because they seemed to only warn, not encourage. I learned to shut out negative messages as best I could and to turn my focus to other things that were more helpful.

I also learned how important it is not to hide from fear, not to deny its existence. This is how I was able to get my courage up for pregnancy and natural birth number two. I was ecstatic to be pregnant a second time when I first found out and then 'poof.' A huge cloud of worry descended over me. A hundred 'what-ifs' (those damn what-ifs do not give up easily). What if the first time I only got lucky? What if my positive karma had run out? What if X, Y and Z worst case scenarios happened? I wanted to be happy and share the news and all I could do was quake with fear. The first pregnancy and birth had gone so well overall that I was afraid I might somehow jinx the second one by even talking about it! No one knew but me, and my current approach wasn't helping me move forward at all, so I got busy. I went out immediately for a stroll and listed off, out loud, every single thing I was afraid of, silly or not, realistic or not, I spewed everything out. That made me feel a lot better, to admit, out loud, what I was afraid of. I didn't want to give my fears too much power by overindulging them, BUT, I also did not want to have my head up my jack-o-lantern by denying that I was a big scared y-cat sometimes.

As D-day (Due-date day) drew closer and closer I increased my resolve to stay focused and to turn away from negativity in all forms, from media, movies, books and even people. By this point I had an almost alarmingly physical reaction to traumatic stories or gory media. It could even sometimes make me nauseous. The link between my body and mind had never been so strong. My yoga teacher was often talking about keeping our diet clean. He wasn't only referring to eating lots of fruits and vegetables but all the things that people consume. He would tell us that watching negativity or drama on TV just for the fun of it was as bad as consuming unhealthy food. Being pregnant put my sensitivity at an all-time high. Working on a positive mindset was the biggest job I had at that point in time.

Just MOVE

"Wait. What? Where are you going?"

The couple walks briskly towards us. I can't help but watch them as they carry their infant towards their car in the parking lot. All three of them look healthy, fit and stunning, and purposeful? I take a breath and gather my nerve. I'm nine months pregnant and desperate to get to the point where they are, out and about feeling great with my newborn. What have I got to lose? "Hi, excuse me. Sorry to bother you but I just wanted to say you guys all look amazing." Did I actually just randomly say that to a stranger? They smile and thank me. My face reddens but I continue anyways: "Any tips?" The woman seems to 'get' me. She was where I was not long ago. She pauses thoughtfully before speaking, noticing my obviously pregnant belly. "You already into fitness?" I nod. Then one word. "Move. Just... Move."

(Moments later)... "Did you seriously just ask a complete stranger for fitness advice?"

"Yup."

"OMG, ha, ha, you're crazy."

(Laughing) "I know!"

I was on the lookout for some encouragement, beyond my midwifery team, and thankfully I did eventually find some. Stories about challenging situations seemed easy to come by but the other variety? Not so much. I needed to find role models who I could relate to and it turned out one was under my very nose. A very good friend, Suzanne, had birthed recently with a midwife without overdue complaint. She told me about what she had done to stay active right until the end of her pregnancy (which had seemed pretty intense even to me at the time). She openly shared the story of her relatively quick labour, her struggles physically and emotionally, in amazingly honest detail. I was moved. I was impressed. Hearing it from word of mouth gave me a little more footing on the idea of a non-medicated birth. I had more hope now. We were of similar age and circumstance. If she had done it maybe I had a good chance too.

I had also been attending fitness classes at my local gym for years and was casually friendly with many of the other regulars and some fitness instructors. I decided to ask them about their experiences and many of these women happily and proudly shared their birthing stories with me. What a 180 degree difference! Suddenly I was hearing very different things, very different outcomes, more in line with my friend Suzanne's story. Short labours, strong but manageable pain, quick recovery times, and the list went on. A lot of them used no pain medication. I particularly remember some instructors and very regular gym attendees telling me that they kept moving, sweating, training their muscles and even teaching until near the end of pregnancy (or comfortably close to it). It gave me new hope, finally people in front of me who had different things to say.

Home Birth

Getting Buy-in

"Can you babysit tonight?"

"I can't, this baby is due any second and I have to keep myself and my house ready."

"So you are saying you won't babysit for me tonight because it is more important to keep your house clean? Seriously?"

"I am saying I just can't, there are a lot of reasons. I am about to have a baby any minute now, I just, oh never mind..."

(Next day) "You haven't called me in days. I need to know what is going on. No one has told me anything. This is not fun for me, I need to be in on things."

"I am sorry, I am in the midst of the final days here and doing my best to stay focused."

"Well, why haven't you called me to update me?"

"Look, I am the one having the baby. (Pause) I know you are worried, so why don't you pick up the phone and call me. I have so much to think about as it is."

"Oh. Um, well, is that what you need, for us to check in with you instead?"

"It is."

"OK."

This part is funny for me to read now, looking back. But not so much so at the time. I've always been more non-confrontational in nature and being clear on boundaries is not, shall we say, second nature. So when I was pregnant I had to learn the hard way how to say no. My extended family was a mixed bag of mostly support with some healthy scepticisms. Unless I felt very close to or supported by a person, I decided to just be rather vague when asked where I planned to give birth, and I didn't even bother telling them much about my birth plans, hopes or dreams. I already knew I wouldn't really feel encouraged and could not afford the emotional energy to get into debates or entertain more fear in any form, even if it was well-intended. Luckily for me it was (and is) still mostly the expected norm that women have babies in hospitals, and everyone in my circle just expected this is what I would also do.

My mother knew my plans and wanted to help me and protect me. In our family the tradition is often to go and hold vigil when someone else is in need. A lovely tradition. *But,* I don't happen to have a cozy waiting room with a separate entrance at my house. I had been very clear that no one was invited to join me when baby time came. So my mother took this request in stride and said she would camp out in my driveway instead. For real.

Another family member would drive back and forth in front of my house 'randomly,' to see if the midwives' cars were in the driveway so she could know when the action started. I had to prepare my midwives to deal with possible door crashers at the last minute. My team was wonderful and had a plan in place to refuse entry to absolutely anyone. I needed nerves of steel to go through this upcoming event and I simply could not afford any extra fear showing up on my driveway or to focus at all on the needs of others. The other part is that frankly, I am just a very private person when it comes to certain things. I was not used to being the centre of attention when I was in pain.

I did run into a few snags with some people in my clan. For starters, some people treated me status quo, like asking me to babysit on my due date. I can see why, since I was not technically *leaving* my place to get the deed done, and they didn't understand that I had to keep my house ready to go.

I learned quickly that a baby can be seen as family property to some. This was going to be the first grandchild or first niece or nephew for some and everyone was excited to be a part of the baby's life. At first I thought it was harmless, sweet and cute. By the third time I had to say 'no' to the same person who insisted on attending the birth I knew I had a sticky mess on my hands. Some people really, *really* wanted to connect with this little thing. I worried that as the mother of the child, the one who needed privacy and space, I didn't filter much into the equation, no matter how many times I explained my needs or wishes. I had to get really loud and clear that I was not okay with guests present and that it wouldn't work for me. In the end my words apparently stung no matter how gentle and loving I tried to be, and they sometimes simply fell on deaf ears. It would take a few years to finally get things back on track and for the dust to settle in a couple of relationships.

One relationship in particular took its toll on me. We had been the best of friends, supporters, and buddies, but parenthood seemed to change everything. I had to draw a very difficult line to insist the person not attend the birth. My request that the baby stay close to me in the early days and that no private videos be shared until I was ready didn't go over well either and were used to turn other family members against me. We both ended up feeling beaten, bruised, and totally misunderstood. She did things so differently and had such a different perspective on what I should be ok with that we seemed miles and miles apart in our views.

For so long people were used to seeing one side of me, and the new, uncertain yet courageous mother coming forward must have been a shock. When people would leave the room or building with my new first born without checking in with me or gaining my confidence first I would feel worried, betrayed, and a pile of other things. It was like someone walking off with part of my body and very, very few people seemed to 'get' that. And I really, really needed to feel 'understood.' Everything was completely new and attachment to my baby was paramount. With each birth my feelings and comfort level would change and by the third round I was much more relaxed and sure of myself, resulting in much less tension for everyone.

In the end, although I found it very disconcerting, I was able to stand my ground and create the boundaries I needed for a peaceful, calm birth. I intuitively believed in birth as a natural process, as something the body is designed to do, even if I didn't quite know how to perfectly articulate that to others yet. I knew somehow that under the right circumstances my body would do whatever it needed to do. One person who never once vacillated in this belief was my yoga teacher. In fact I would leave the class feeling encouraged and capable, even on days when a sense of hopelessness or fear had seemed to creep in. Thankfully I also had my very small inner circle of people, including my husband and Suzette, who thought I could handle it the way I wanted to and never wavered in their conviction or support.

First Birth

This was my dark night of the soul. This was me being tested, on every possible level. My endurance, my threshold for pain, my determination and my faith in spirit, in myself and everything else.

We are still all alone, but this is the least of my worries. Shouldn't our midwife have returned to us by now? My birth partner is getting more stressed. I, meanwhile, don't care all that much that we are alone. I am not worried about it, I am more worried about making it through, staying awake, surviving this avalanche of pain. I just need to navigate through this. We can catch the baby ourselves if we absolutely have to, I am quite certain of it.

This is bigger, more serious and crazier to navigate than I could have expected. I am trying to follow my body's orders without getting completely knocked overboard. I am trying to not be too scared. I am truly surprised at the level of discomfort that has spread through the majority of my body, every nerve echoing the ferocious energy of the contractions moving through me. I think I have done everything I can think of to be prepared, except get enough rest that evening. I have tried in my way to create a body and mindset as strong as I could to provide balance amidst the storm around and within me. I have worked and trained for weeks if not years to prepare myself for this day, haven't I? How absolutely bad could it be? Is this what a marathon is like towards the end? I'll take the marathon any day, at least by now I would have the option to be walking.

My partner diligently takes the time measurements between contractions. Two minutes. Three minutes. One and a half minutes. Skip a minute. Back to two minutes. Dammit. There seems to be no clear pattern to us novice time keepers, and we are dutifully waiting for time between sensations to be very consistent before calling our midwife again but consistency never comes. We have no way of knowing that my natural labouring pattern will never be specific to the minute, that that is just the way my body works. After two hours of keeping track I am getting frustrated with it. Soon we can no longer keep track of the time measurements, everything is happening so close together and it's all just becoming one big blur.

My entire body is literally roaring to life and poised, every single inch of it directed towards a specific goal. I can almost sense the precision and perfect alignment of what is happening inside of me but I'm really in way too much pain and too overwhelmed by it to care. My nervous system and every nerve everywhere commands my 100% full attention. My skin is beyond hypersensitive to the touch. I'm hot and I'm cold. My voice still works, miraculously, though it takes great effort to talk now.

My body is completely doing its own thing, it's as though I am one huge ball of sensation, of pain, and all I can do is keep breathing and allowing. I am not in charge anymore. I am acutely present yet not at the same time. It's all surreal. I know the baby is about to be born. My partner is even more panicked now... I keep breathing... he asks me to please hold on until the midwife arrives. Yeah right, as if I had any say in the matter. I couldn't hold this process back if I tried, it's like I just need to not fight the sensations and allow them to do their work, even though this is very hard to do. With whatever ounce of voice I can muster I try to reassure him that everything will be fine. I realize I have to totally surrender the fight and drop my gloves.

At first it all just seemed like a crazy waiting game. I had made sure to book off work a few weeks early to keep myself healthy and mentally fit. My new manager at work questioned my request to leave early and I had to provide a note from my care provider.

Because my midwives had assured me that it was normal for a first pregnancy to go beyond 40 weeks and that mine likely would do so, I knew not to panic when my 41st week rolled around. I was, however, starting to get more uncomfortable and annoyed and worried about when things would get rolling. I just wanted to meet this person, wanted everything to be done with, wanted a safe delivery, and wanted to sleep well again (ha, ha, ha, boy, I *really* had no clue). On my due date I celebrated the day by taking a long nature hike. I remember putting aside my sadness and worries about how much longer the pregnancy would be for a few moments on the trail and thinking that there was no other way I would rather be spending my day. I had to accept that this baby would just take as long as it needed and so be it.

The day of the birth started like the rest, me feeling mostly fine, (for a 41-and-a-half-week pregnant woman) optimistic and hopeful, and scared of the unknown, all rolled into one. I had tried my best to give up expectations and predicting when the baby would arrive (although by this point I secretly began to wonder if it ever would). I woke up and immediately drank lots of room temperature water (an ingrained habit I learned from my yoga teacher), did whatever stretches and movement I felt up to, performed my breathing exercises, ate oatmeal and a kale smoothie and went for a long, long walk (Yup, I really had that much freedom and energy to put towards my self-care back then, sigh.). I walked even longer and further than my usual daily treks. It was mid-August, a nice warm sunny day. I made my way to a field I had never explored before.

I paused in the middle of the field, crouched down and touched the earth, and in the silence of my natural surroundings took a moment to genuinely tune into what I was feeling: anticipation, frustration, impatience, fear, hope, excitement and everything in-between. Closing my eyes I asked my body and baby to *please* move to the next stage. I was teary-eyed by the time I arrived home. I thought about anything else I could do to encourage this baby to move its butt on out, so to speak. A thought struck: why not write a letter? So I sat alone on the back porch and wrote my heart out, about how I was totally ready to hold my little one in my arms, how it was safe to come out, how everyone wanted to meet him or her. I cried and cried and wrote from the heart. I have never shown anyone this letter. I am saving it so my child can read it when the time is right. After I finished I felt relieved and could breathe deeply and peacefully and let it all go.

I lied down for a nap mid-afternoon. I was already in almost daily contact with my midwife (as is the norm in late pregnancy) but I hadn't called her yet that day. I don't know if I actually slept but I awoke to my water breaking. Yes! Finally! I was delighted to get this show on the road. Our midwife joined us after dinner and we sat chatting for hours about what was to come and what could be an issue. She explained the time-lines we were looking at. If we wanted the baby to come at home it needed to come by morning, preferably. No problem, I thought! I felt happy, scared, confident, and really excited to finally meet and hold the new person. I agreed to an internal sweep (to get things moving, just in case) and drinking some castor oil (also to get things moving, just in case). Our midwife left our home around 11:30 at night, telling us she expected to likely return to us near dawn. In her experience first time mothers took longer in the early stages of labour and she thought I would take at least all night to go through it. We told her we'd call her when the contractions were strong and steady and consistent, as she requested we do. When she left I was feeling strong cramps, but being inexperienced, didn't realize I was already well into labour. And as it turned out, this was not going to take until dawn.

The first hour we danced a little. I remember crying softly, releasing a pent up wall of emotion that the time was *finally* upon us, feeling happy, scared and somewhat electrified at the prospect of what I now had to face. I would finally get to meet this person face to face yet there was a ways to go. We sat on our meditation mats for a long while and slowly breathed, staying very calm and centred. The intensity of the sensations I was feeling increased gradually until I could no longer sit down, and wouldn't even consider lying down. I discovered I needed to stay upright or on my hands and knees to navigate the pain and take the full body breaths I needed. Using castor oil? It turns out it was unnecessary in my opinion, same thing with the sweep. The oil made me nauseous. Being sick while also being in labour: not-much-fun-at-all. But I got through it. Looking back I realize one of my biggest challenges besides the pain of the contractions was my level of fatigue. No point here having a "coulda-woulda-shoulda" discussion I realize, but still, if only I had rested more, stayed laying down all evening instead of up talking and tidying the house and getting things ready and whatever else I was doing. Hindsight is 20-20.

I stayed in the warm shower in table top pose for what felt like forever. I eventually got out because I was worried I would run out of hot water. By now it was closer to 2:00 am, I had found an upright position leaning into some comfy pillows that was as comfortable as possible and the sensations were getting bigger and bigger every few minutes. I remembered to keep swaying and gentling moving in whatever way my body wanted to and stayed focused on working with my breath. One breath blended into the next one for an eternity. One wave of pain would crash upon me and then there would be none for a few minutes. This seemed to go one forever. We called my midwife. She felt I wasn't close to birth yet. You see I think the problem with me is that, my voice sounds steady and I appear to not be in pain EVEN WHEN I AM. Having never had a baby before, however, I couldn't argue much and agreed to call her back when things picked up. The sensations became closer and closer over the next hour (by this point I was vacillating between almost falling asleep in between contractions and breathing through the worst pain of my life on the other).

When things were happening at an even faster tempo we called the midwife once again. Our midwife still doubted my late labour stage, (guess I still sounded calm and I could easily speak, good to know that I can hold a conversation even when in so much pain I want to keel over). Luckily, however, she stayed on the phone for a while, heard me go through a contraction and then immediately told us she'd be right over. By the time she arrived I was lost on a sea of painful waves crashing every few seconds, it was almost surreal. I could do nothing but surrender and let things roll through me. I kept breathing slowly and deeply. I was present yet not at the same time. There were times, during this labour, I just wanted out, I just wanted to get far away from the pain. I had never experienced anything like this, especially for a prolonged period of time. I'll be real. I was completely shocked at first and taken aback by it. Yes I had 'read' and conceptually understood this is 50 times worse than what you'd expect but still!

My other half was *not* relaxed about the idea of delivering a baby himself at that point in time. When our midwife finally came to my side the baby was crowning, and I am sure he almost melted with relief. She quickly put on a pair of gloves and told my husband to run to the car for her other supplies. I could see he was visibly torn, not wanting to leave me (I remember asking him not to leave). He rushed out to her car and couldn't find the right bag. He had to go back and forth once or twice more, probably the fastest footsteps he had ever taken. He made it back in time. The midwife had me adjust my breathing as she carefully added some gentle counter-pressure to help avoid tearing. I was already *way* past being able to take any more of this situation when the burning feeling briefly intensified even more. And then, boom, the full-sized baby made her appearance with a single protesting squeak and the dog, confused at the new voice in the home, started barking in reply. Then very suddenly, finally, all was silent and still for a moment.

I could barely catch my breath, in complete shock, *what the hell just happened to me?* Suddenly I'm fine, I am totally fine. No more pain. No more fear. It's really, really over after all this time and I get to hold the baby. I could have collapsed into a puddle of relief. But no, within a split second my attention went 100% to the baby. My adrenaline and energy levels shot through the roof. I picked up the beautiful, large, long, alert, calm baby in front of me and I would never put her down again. She blinked her eyes once or twice. I was smiling. I was shaking. Was I also crying? *No, I don't want to sit down I really am feeling fine being upright. No, seriously, I just want to stay in this spot holding her.* It was about 4:00 am. The whole active labour had been about four and a half hours long. Accomplishment, *relief* and awe overcame me. I never knew gratitude, really, like I did in those moments. For everything and everyone around me. The greatest moment of my life had just flashed before me. It would change me inside-out for years to come.

Aftermath

There is a long silence while I collapse into tears awaiting their judgement on my fate. Having an examination after everything I just went through should be no big deal. I have been feeling great until this point, yet I am suddenly quite solemn. Somehow I would rather go through it all again than face a needle and thread. I just want to leave my body alone and to start to collect myself again. I visualize a positive result with all my might yet also resign myself to the inevitable and gather my courage like a cloak around me.

And then I hear the words, "You know, she'll be fine actually. We don't even need to do any repair work. Wow, I can't believe what you got away with as a first timer and with such a big full-sized baby."

Me, silently: "Thank you, thank you, thank you, thank you, thank you, thank you, thank you, thank you, thank you, thank you, thank you, thank you, thank you, thank you, thank you."

Our second midwife, Rachel, arrived shortly after the birth. This was unusual as midwives usually work in teams but in my case things happened more quickly than expected. I was not breaking my physical connection with the baby and did not put her down, even when they insisted I use the bathroom. Rachel told me it was highly unconventional to bring a baby with me but smiled permissively at the same time. That was the beginning of my inner warrior coming through into motherhood. My helpers were surprised by my steadiness on my feet. They eventually convinced me to lay down, even though I didn't really feel the need to do so. I was still feeling like I was full of energy and wide awake. My aftermath examination was positive, thank the lord! (And maybe the high vitamin E content sesame oil?) The level of gratitude and empowerment I felt was insane. I was so in the mood to celebrate and was now so very happy to have my whole midwife team around us to share in the joy.

A third midwife arrived. Everyone helped with all the standard procedures such as weighing the baby, checking our blood pressure, cutting the cord, etc. I loved that my baby was administered to while she was nursing which took tons of stress off my shoulders. The midwives were there taking care of us and cleaning everything up for a few hours before they tucked us all snuggly into bed and promised to return the next day. I still felt euphoric and could barely sleep.

The remainder of that night and the following day was one of, if not the, best day of my life. Perhaps it's because of the crazy oxytocin rush your body receives after giving birth, or perhaps it was simply because I was so very relieved to be done with the process and all the waiting and worry beforehand. It may have also been because all my focus was now on the little angel in my arms. There was also the fire that was now lit in me that had to do with facing something terrifying and coming out of it on the other end. I felt very proud for listening to my instincts and not nursing everyone's fears, including my own. My daughter was nursing like a champ and gained weight every day. We were a team, we had climbed this crazy challenging mountain together and nothing would be the same again.

I somehow didn't expect anything from anyone, yet one of my sisters rushed over with a small balloon and some flowers and offered to go to the store for me. Another sister brought me some muffins she had made and a big yellow smiley happy face balloon, which still brings tears to my eyes. My parents came next with a lovely baby basket and nursing pillow and tons of love, and my in-laws sent a bouquet and loving messages. I was so very touched by these little gifts and offerings. More like blown away. I really had not been expecting anything as I had been so focused on getting through the birth I had not stopped to think about how I might want to celebrate it afterwards.

Taking Time to Recover

I suddenly fell in love with my body and its abilities. That may sound strange, and indeed I remember thinking it was very strange myself, but the second I gave birth I literally saw my body in a totally new way and I actually felt it looked better than it ever had. It certainly seemed stronger than it ever had. My midwife was adamant that I needed to take it easy and rest at least for a week, and not do anything strenuous, even if I felt like I could do so (which I did). *Why do you think so many of those women in previous centuries were dying and bleeding out after the babies were born? Post-partum hemorrhaging is a real and serious thing!*

Both my partner and I took recovery seriously.

I have to say that the convenience and comfort of midwives attending me at home was superb. They arrived early each of the two mornings after the birth, and then again during the day after that. They took great care of me and went through all the follow-up questions and procedures without me even having to leave my cozy bed. They were gentle and sympathetic and helpful with just about everything, even offering to tidy the kitchen. They gave me all the breastfeeding support and encouragement I could have wanted or needed. I was surprised at how comfortable I felt in their presence. Our primary midwife came back to visit us at home several more times the first week to make sure all was going well. She took hours to teach us how to properly wrap a baby in a sling and to give us tips and advice on dealing with gas, burping and getting a baby to fall asleep at night.

When it came time for the baby's first blood test (a heel prick) I was nervous and loath to hurt her. I wanted to nurse her but at the time I just wasn't ready to stand by or watch while the procedure was done so I went and hid in the next room. My midwife made me feel better by telling me that she herself had had to go hide and block out the sound using the shower when her own child had her first blood drawn.

The baby's demeanour and expression shifted as she watched me leave the room. Two days old but she could readily sense my anxiety and knew something was up. She was held gently over my spouse's shoulder while our midwife pricked her heel. Not enough blood coming out. She had to try again. The little one was distressed and crying loudly by now. So I took a breath, womaned-up, and took her in my own arms. I was so grateful I did. She settled a little more and things went smoothly this second time around. We went through it together like we had done everything else.

Overall, I focused on the baby while cooking up some awesome plant-based meals, drank plenty of lemon water with pressed ginger, and was ordered to rest most of the time. When we took the baby for her first short walk on day three Vince insisted shortly after lift-off that I turn around and go back home. I laughed at the idea of only going for a four minute walk but didn't argue. He was following our midwives' orders to the T. Finally after a week I started to go for longer walks but hadn't actually gone anywhere else yet. I remember anxiously and very tentatively trying a single sun salutation about 6 days after the birth. I was nervous, but crazy curious to see what it would feel like to move within what felt like a brand new body. Would my muscles hold up? Would it feel completely different than before? Would I have *any* core strength left whatsoever? I was very pleasantly surprised to see that everything worked exactly as it had before. Actually, it was like I had never been pregnant at all. It was easy to move, and it seemed like my muscles hadn't lost any of their strength. As instructed I avoided ab work or anything strenuous for quite some time, knowing I needed a few more weeks for the uterus to shift itself back to its normal size.

Afterthoughts

My labour progressed really nicely and quickly and I feel this was due to several things. One, I stayed upright then mostly in table top position (hands and knees or leaning forward over some cushions) and two, I felt I had all the privacy I needed and was comfortable in my own domain. I am just not good with being in pain around other people. It completely distracts me on a lot of levels. I know it may sound weird but I was completely okay with my midwife not being present until the end of my first labour (although my partner, a first-timer himself that night, likely has his own different views). Technically I could have insisted my midwife come sooner, but I just didn't know how far along I was yet so I let her be the judge of when to come. I wasn't seriously worried about the physical process somehow. I think at the time privacy was a huge concern for me and I simply sensed that I was best left in my own bubble and that things would be best that way.

The only serious concern I had outside of managing the contractions was my level of fatigue. I had forgotten that it is a natural part of the hormonal birthing process to feel deeply tired between contractions.

During certain moments in labour I felt overwhelmed, abandoned, depleted, and at the end of my rope in every single way possible. And this was while I was in my own room with nice candles lit and a gentle, safe ambiance all around me. I cannot imagine having accomplished this for the first time under other circumstances. Talk about getting to know oneself!

As the days after the birth wore on real life gradually sunk in and the realities of parenting for the first time obliviated everything else. It was a happy time and an exhausting time. More family came to visit immediately for a few days (this is before I knew how much space I needed to rest and rejuvenate after a big event). And my better half, god bless him, still on vacation from work, got busy ripping up the carpets and hammering away putting in hard wood floors. Yup. With a newborn in the house.

I remember being amused and annoyed when one family member lectured me late one evening just after having the baby. I had just gotten the baby to sleep and knew she would wake back up for a feeding in another hour. I decided to dive into a nice big juicy piece of chocolate cake as a little treat. I hadn't taken but one bite when I heard, "...tsk, tsk, tsk, you shouldn't be eating dessert before bed because you won't sleep well tonight." Did you just say that to a mom who just gave birth? Really? He's lucky he didn't get the chocolate cake in the head.

Instead I took my cake up to my room and enjoyed it in privacy. I know, I know, everyone means well and has good intentions. I truly believe that. But sometimes... well you just need to be left alone to have your cake and eat it too.

By now I was needing to rest and just have some me time and focus on what I needed without feeling the pressure of guests, yet another family member came down to stay with us right away for a few weeks. On the one hand I was very grateful for the company and the extra help around the house, even as I also struggled with our very different parenting approaches and trying to put my own needs and boundaries in the open for the first time. I very much needed to do things my own way and stay very connected to my child, and at the same time was deeply worried about hurting anyone's feelings. Plus everything was totally new. Nursing every other hour kept me very busy and I had no energy for even very subtle confrontation. It was still scary to say 'no.' I would get better at this with time.

Everyone seemed to have different opinions about everything. A lot of my family and friends couldn't have cared less about our choices, a few were skeptical but respectful, and about 2% were scandalized. Within a month I received a completely random phone call from a distant relative I had only ever talked to once or twice before. She was crystal clear and dove right in by saying, "I think the whole problem with babies not sleeping *through* the night lies with the mother, it's the mother that's the issue." *So nice to hear from you! And I do have a baby that sleeps through the whole night, she just wakes up for milk several times in the process.* The out of the blue criticism stung yet I knew I couldn't win the war and had no energy to fight it. Doing things 'differently' was hardly a new label for me to wear. I realize now her beliefs and perspectives are her own just as mine are my own.

As the days wore on I learned gradually more and more about the world of parenting an infant. I spent a lot of time sitting outside doing pranayama with the baby in my lap and taking long walks with her snuggled on me in a carrier. I enjoyed these moments and made the best I could out of this new way of life. It would be a long time before I would think about gearing myself up to do the whole thing again. I eventually found my way to a mom and baby yoga class. Ahhh. There were all sorts of other moms, other birth-at-home moms, and moms who worked with midwives, and now my clan would grow and change for the better.

Birth #2, Healing the Scars

Hands down, one of the best days, moments and memories of my life. What can I say? Looking at those last words, I know it sounds hard to believe, especially based on what I once believed about birth. But don't let me fool you. This doesn't mean it was easy, or that it wasn't enormously challenging and that I didn't get well-prepared first.

Throughout this pregnancy I became more and more aware of the idea that you *can* get ready for birth and improve the odds of things being easier to manage. But I still had lots of internal house cleaning to do. I realized after my first child was born that, even though I had no physical scars, I was still resentful somehow. I had been stunned and very disappointed by the amount of pain I had experienced. It had shocked me somewhat. I don't know if I had naïvely hoped that birth would be more comfortable than it was or that I would be somehow exempted from serious labour pain by practicing healthy living or what. But it was a real feeling. I was scarred emotionally from the experience for some months.

During the more intense moments of labour I had felt completely betrayed, ravaged and 100% abandoned. Nothing was arriving to save me from the agony I was in. Emotional and energetic healing sessions that came much later would confirm the trauma that was imprinted in me due to this labour. I won't sugar-coat what felt like brief moments of torture, you can't get away from, feeling like you can't get through it no matter how strong you are and you think you might even want to die because of it. When women say, 'I can't do this,' boy do I get that now. It was traumatic and psychologically scarring. I didn't think I'd get to a point where I would say, 'I can't do this,' or at least I sure as hell hoped I *would* not get to that point. But I did. And my birth partner totally expected it and was able to stay the course emotionally and not panic alongside me when I said it.

But then here's the thing, how can I easily go on to tell you that, poof, literally from the second the baby was out of my body and I picked her up, there was no more pain, no more fatigue, no more fear, no more anything but love and joy and insane energy currents everywhere. I felt indestructible. I felt strong. I didn't want to or need to 'lie down' or 'take Tylenol' and really didn't understand why they kept suggesting it. Take it for what? The hell of it? Stop with the pills already I don't want them and don't need them.

Gradually, with patience and the help of a healer and my own wellness practices I processed the brunt of the trauma and came to a place where I could face embracing that pain much more easily.

Over time, the fear of birth pain did not completely disappear but it did become more of a partnership than a dictatorship. My midwives assured me that second births are typically faster and less painful than the first. (And thank heavens for that.)

This pregnancy felt a little different. I sensed a different kind of energy with this baby, more of a serene quietness. Whereas with the other pregnancies I was craving movement and music, during this one I was more drawn inward and spent more time in quietness and contemplation, in meditation and just being more connected with my spiritual side. For my baby shower a good friend came to lead all us women in belly dancing and we did a blessing way. A blessing way was a new tradition for me in which each woman presents the pregnant mother with a blessing and then gives a bead to put on a necklace that can be worn during or around birth. I was deeply moved by the energy in the blessings we received. One of my friends, Rachelle, is a poet and between her beautifully crafted verses and everyone else's beautiful words we were all nice and teary-eyed.

As my due date drew nearer I once again decided to leave a few weeks early to take care of my pregnancy and prepare myself for birth. It was over 18 months since my last baby had been born. Though the local birthing centre was now open, I decided to go ahead with home birth again. After the first experience I just saw it as a perfect, natural and convenient fit for me. I knew that if I had to go through something that painful again, home was where I wanted it to happen.

The waiting game is a really suspenseful rollercoaster ride. Despite knowing that it's very normal and to be expected that babies come later (or earlier sometimes) than the commonly prescribed 40 weeks, it was still hard to not really want the baby to come 'on time' or just a teeny bit early. I would feel totally confident and happy and unworried about the delivery date and then slip into worrying that something was taking too long, or maybe something wasn't right within a matter of hours. It did cause anxiousness and fretfulness and was very, very annoying sometimes. I had no desire to know 'exactly when' as it wouldn't feel natural for me, but on the other hand waiting for a signal of impending birth was like sitting at the front door with your snowsuit and hats and mitts and boots and backpack and starting to break a sweat, all ready to go but you don't know when the bus is going to show up!

After waiting for what seemed like ages for this little soul to present himself (when in fact he was just a little over a week late, same as the others), I finally felt some gentle contractions early one morning after doing my morning exercises (yup, I was still able to squeeze my yoga routine into my schedule at that point, but not for long). The rest of the family had still been sleeping. I spent the day very peacefully, eating vegetable stew, (like other big stressful events or workouts, I felt better about going into childbirth with less food in my belly, and also purposefully avoided any inflammatory foods that day), walking and even napping lightly during some very light contractions. I did not want to go into final stage labour already tired from a busy day as I had the first time around.

By about 4 pm we asked the midwife to pop by. I was crying as I opened the door to welcome her. She looked concerned. I explained I was crying not because of pain but because it was the first time I had ever had to send my daughter away for a lengthy period of time (to a trusted female friend who lived nearby). It turned out I was only in the early stages of labour. My plan was therefore to send my midwife home to her own children. My protective birth partner objected as he had no desire to go through the event almost alone again. Also our midwife, Rachel, had attended as a back-up at my first birth and knew I was a very silent type who could transition quite quickly, so she stayed.

Birth pains intensified gradually. This time round I could really calmly and clearly see how the amount of attention I was paying to my labour increased its progress. The friend babysitting my daughter was wonderful and sent me pictures so I could relax and not worry about how my daughter was doing. But my friend had small children of her own and it would only be a matter of time before my daughter needed me. So I made up my mind, I was ready and this baby had to come sooner than later. By about 6:00 pm I was in a whole lot of pain, on and off, and determined to stay on my feet to encourage delivery. Rachel granted us plenty of privacy and we tucked ourselves away in a separate room and put on some relaxing music. I cried softly for the pain I was feeling and especially for the pain that was to come as I slowly continued to build my nerve up for the actual birth. I was scared, I was letting myself feel it and kept turning towards the event instead of away from it. I felt like I was literally walking straight into it, calmly and with dignity. Very fearful yet also determined and accepting. I had already dropped my gloves on this one and I was letting the birth process take over here on out.

We continued to walk gently or we just swayed together on the spot, over and over. I stayed on my feet, moving in whatever way felt comfortable, for as long as I possibly could and would lean on my partner or on a piece of furniture when a contraction rolled around. I had done lots of research on natural pain relief and decided to try some Ayurveda rolling techniques, applying pressure to birthing points along the wrists and forearms using a small roller. I feel that it helped speed things up. Whether it did or not, it certainly was a nice distraction from the onslaught of waves starting to hit faster and harder. I would be startled and struggling through a particularly painful moment when my partner asked if he should stop the rolling. "No," I almost snapped. I found the rhythmic motion reassuring and it gave me a small anchor in the storm to hold onto.

As things sped up and the pain increased in intensity I silently wondered how on earth I was going to survive this situation again. I prayed, I repeated affirmations silently and did everything I could think of to help this birth be shorter and not as painful as the last one.

Rachel was now in our company but stayed blissfully and respectfully quiet while lending us her presence and silent reassurance. She was listening to my breathing for signs of progress and would occasionally put the stethoscope gently on my belly to check the baby's heart rate. It was nice and steady.

I kept up the very long deep breathing, *especially* during the contractions. They would start mildly then reach an almost crazy painful crescendo point before lessening to almost nothing. Over and over I hit them head-on and kept my breathing steady through the buildup, the peak of the wave, then the decrescendo back to neutral. I questioned why I was so drugged with this sudden feeling of sleepiness between contractions, like someone had actually given me some sort of sleeping pill type of feeling. Rachel explained that my body, via my hormones, was purposefully giving me a break and to relax while I could and take advantage of the sleepy feeling. (Wish I had known that the first time around!) So, instead of the fatigue making me alarmed I let myself slip into a cozy cocoon of almost sleeping between the contractions. They were still very painful, but nowhere near like it was with the first birth. I was very, very focused. More than ever. And I was scared and felt helpless and vulnerable too. I was inching closer and closer to a feeling of desperation and panic which never really overtook me when the ending came even faster than I'd hoped.

My body had totally taken over and then seemingly out of nowhere it reared up for one super long powerful pushing sensation. Poof. Halfway there. My body was already in the midst of a second heroic-sized push before I even realized it (I really kind of felt like a witness and as though I wasn't going through it) and just like that the baby was born. I was still in my upright position when I leaned down to take the baby from the midwife's hands. I had burst into tears, we all did actually! All I could say was, "Thank you, thank you, thank you," over and over again.

Peeking more consciously at my environment I suddenly realized it has grown dark, the room gently aglow in candlelight. Through my tears I hadn't realized that the baby was looking a tad dark in colour as I was holding him a little sideways. I set him up higher with his feet towards the floor and his colour normalized. He was gorgeous, and… a boy! We never found out the gender of our babies until they were born. I was hoping for a boy this time round and here he was. The four of us just sort of sat and smiled and laughed and cried for a few minutes while I caught my breath. Active labour for only about three hours. Two pushes. Whaaaaat? I was totally stunned, in awe of what had just happened and once again a serious sense of empowerment and gratitude swept through me. I was also melting with relief that it was over, finally, and was just eager to enjoy the new addition.

The back-up midwives didn't make it in time. I was 100% okay with that and lovingly yet openly told them afterward that I secretly preferred it that way. I can sense other people's energy around me and am easily distracted by it. I tend to feel self-conscious when I am in pain and therefore don't relax as well. I had created a deep place of being centred when in labour. Rachel, God bless her, had been the perfect birth companion for me. Leaving us alone unless necessary, to move and be in the zone in quiet and stillness. I am so grateful for her peaceful calmness. She is born to do what she does!

Once again, the midwives went through all the follow-up procedures with us, made sure I was doing well, baby was nursing and doing great, cleaned everything up, tucked us into bed and promised to be back in the morning to check in. My older daughter came back home to me around 10:00 pm. I was concerned about how she might, at 18 months old, receive seeing a baby sibling in her mother's arms. We had discussed all sorts of scenarios and had different plans for how to introduce her to her brother, but in the end I just took the direct route. I had him in my arms when she toddled into the room. Thankfully she took it well. She didn't actually seem overly concerned by the new addition, she simply asked to nurse (which was awesome because it helped bring the milk in faster for the newborn), and then went to bed. It had been a very big, life changing day and I could not wait to share the news. I was bursting with joy and was proud at having completed something that terrified me once again, straight on. I ordered a favourite treat to celebrate while we called everyone to say they had a grandson and nephew. I was given a loving yet disapproving frown in response to a request for a specific meal after the birth. One second later, make that one raised annoyed eyebrow from me later, he was out the door and on his way to Tim Hortons. I just went through labour! Give me my damn bagel and cream cheese with a French vanilla already!

Walking directly into labour, without retreating or letting nervousness get the upper hand, took all the courage I never knew I had. There were still moments this time around when it felt like I was completely abandoned to suffer, completely baffled and completely out of control in every possible sense of the word. I would even have a repeat dream later on about having to go into labour again and having to drum up the courage and mental energy to do so. It felt like I was purposely walking into a fire. It really seemed counterintuitive to open up and go along with a situation I knew would be painful. I was able to sit with it and even when it threatened to overwhelm me, it somehow didn't. I used my breathing practices for all they were worth. And it worked. I was so grateful I had felt more ready and had some previous experience this time around.

Home Birth

Birth #3, Putting It All Together

The biggest difference between this birth and the previous two was that I journeyed through a lot of the beginning of the process alone (physically that is, my family and midwife were in the home with me but not in my personal space much at all). The chief reason for this was that as usual, my first born was quite resistant to going to sleep when we most wanted her to. This did not seem to bother me. By now I was steady on my birthing legs. Really, overall, I cannot complain, I really can't. This was and remains one of the most magical evenings of my life and was an incredibly empowering experience for me and I think for my team of midwives as well. But I had better start at the beginning.

Throughout this pregnancy, still on hiatus from my desk job, I was teaching yoga for pregnant women and dance for new mothers while their babies were snuggled into carriers. I got to dance and encourage women to stay active every week, and I felt right at home with a big pregnant belly while doing so. This was so different from the previous pregnancies when I spent a lot more time in a standard fitness setting. I was with lovely women and their new babies and they seemed to delight in their teacher having an ever growing belly on display while she danced.

I also taught some adult yoga classes and I remember late in my seventh month asking the class how they were doing. One gentleman in the back row, out of breath, laughingly said, "Good, but when are you supposed to be slowing down?" I took it as a compliment. It felt great to be teaching others and staying active at the same time. I remember it as a very happy, inspiring time in my life. Because I was also very busy with two toddlers I didn't have all that much time to worry or be anxious about my pregnancy. So different from how I felt the first time around!

Though overall I felt well and healthy, the first months of this pregnancy would see me dealing with some annoying constant morning indigestion and some serious fatigue that would force me to re-prioritize where I was using my energy. Late one evening I was sitting and feeling very worn out, rather like a used sock, and remember complaining and insisting out loud that, no matter what, this winter season I wanted to get somewhere where there would be warmth, sunlight and the ability to go for a walk outside. Seemed simple enough? How I would organize a trip with two toddlers while being in my first trimester I didn't know. I am still stunned at what came next, and yes this is a true story!

Late the very next night, I was getting ready for bed and heard a business conversation going on.

Seemed pretty late for a work call. Within moments the door to the room burst open: "XYZ Company wants to fly us to Turks and Caicos for work. We can all go but we have to leave within two days!" Highly annoyed, knowing this obviously had to be a joke, I shut the door and insisted my emotions not be toyed with. Well, it wasn't a joke, and within two days we were off for some beautiful sunshine and white sands. I have been trying to repeat my secret manifesting formula ever since!

Late in this pregnancy the whole family modified our diet for a few weeks to address a skin condition my child was coping with. I had never gone without sugar or dairy or corn for more than three weeks. I had already been a vegetarian for years and was used to being caffeine-free and wheat-free, but not so religiously, so I found the restrictions to be a challenge at first. Emotionally that is. But physically? It was amazing. Once we had a solid menu in place my sugar cravings dropped almost completely. Not a single meltdown from any children over the whole three weeks. I couldn't believe how good I felt and how much my energy improved. I was not mentally or emotionally ready to maintain the eating style long-term but did keep a lot of the principles in place as much as possible. The process opened my eyes to just how much I lean on foods and sugar for comfort, and what is possible when I step away from those habits and patterns.

The Labour Game

"We are super excited. Due date is tomorrow. And if baby doesn't come we will induce."

"Wait, what, why? Lots of pregnancies go beyond 40 weeks, mine were all nearly 42 weeks..."

"Really? Strange. Well, it's stressful to wait, we don't want to worry."

As my due date approached we lined up two or three trusted people to come over and sit with our children during the night or who could watch them elsewhere if labour occurred during the day. The problem was, of course, the ever-present undeterminable variable: you never know exactly when the baby is going to be born or how long labour will be. My dance with labour started two weeks before I actually gave birth. I had never really experienced Braxton Hicks contractions much, let alone a full-on false start labour. Just before my due date, I went into early labour (or so I thought) and started to get everything ready and in order. The children were asleep, so we set up the living room with an extra bed and mattress and covers and pillows and everything else we might need. My midwife was on standby and I told her I would call her when contractions started getting closer together. I started to walk slowly, sinking into my zone, working with my breath and encouraging things to move along, *for almost the entire night!* Whoops. When morning came the contractions disappeared and I was exhausted. And confused.

This happened a second time after that. I was sure labour was starting and it would proceed for a few hours and then 'poof,' nothing. After the second and third time this happened I got a little fed up with wondering if every twinge was the labour beginning. I remember on my due date just giving up on the whole waiting game. I was tired of it and feeling fed up. I decided to do a great low impact aerobics video called Caribbean Workout and then afterwards loaded up my two toddlers in their double-Bob sports stroller to go for a long walk to get a tea and do some shopping. I was, at that point, tired of waiting and was like, 'whatever, it will happen when it happens.'

As was the case with the first two pregnancies, and as my midwives had always ensured could and would likely happen, my pregnancy was over 40 weeks long (they were all about 41.5 weeks long actually). I am aware this is now accepted as within normal range. But still! I would spend so much time hoping and praying and getting psyched for things to happen on or at least near my due date and then poof! It's like having Christmas with no Santa.

Two days before I actually had my third child I was climbing into a seat and suddenly felt a sharp deep pain in my lower right abdomen. It was isolated and confused me. Was this labour? No, it felt like it had to do with a muscle or ligament. I called my physiotherapist, but she couldn't see me for a few more days. I showed up for my scheduled midwife appointment that day in tears, anxious and miserable overall. I could barely move about since my belly muscles hurt so much. It was hard to be forced to be so still and slow and relatively immobile. I did, however, intuitively believe that these things, especially signs from my body, needed listening to and just maybe my body needed me to be still at that time to prepare. So I was.

The day I gave birth I just needed to get out of the house and convinced my better half to take me and the kids on an outing so I could meet my good friend for tea and a chat. She watched me waddling into the store very slowly and very carefully, taking tiny steps (so I wouldn't irritate my pulled stomach muscle), and laughingly asked if I was ready to pop. Funny how people assume that a pregnancy waddle is due to the weight of the baby. I was moving in the tiniest increments, like a snail, and through my discomfort I was at least able to laugh at myself. Luckily for me I got to sit still while we had a nice distracting chat about the comings and goings in her life. I forgot about my own discomfort while I sipped my tea and listened to her amusing stories.

Then it was time to go home. We were all sort of in 'hover' mode at that point, knowing labour could start at any moment but still wanting to keep things as 'normal' as possible. It was getting annoying to be constantly ready just in case. I once again *had* to have a tidy home to birth in or I just couldn't feel centred or relaxed. Luckily the one thing I could do easily was crawl around on all fours, because that was how I cleaned up my living room area that night. I tried not to be resentful as the rest of the family sat happily watching a show while I went about making sure everything was in order. I guess I really didn't want to sit still anyways. I was restless, tired and at the end of my emotional rope. I had had it with all the false labour starts and was frustrated and sad all at once.

I eventually found solitude and cried and cried, totally exasperated, in pain and generally feeling like crap. What on earth was taking this baby so long? Why all the false starts and this deeply annoying muscle pain hindering my ability to move about? I just wanted to be alone for a while. Gradually I centred myself and some calmness settled over me. I knew that being on all fours puts the baby in an ideal position for birth, so I leaned over my bed and took some needed breaths in silence. I then suddenly remembered a holistic yoga teacher who taught that the downward dog pose can help bring on labour when the time was at hand. So I gently and slowly moved back and forth from cat-cow to downward dog, flowing from one pose to the next, over and over and over again, for a long time. I matched my breath to the motion and continued to move slowly and rhythmically. I stayed alone for some time doing this. And then finally right when I decided I could use a group hug, I got one.

My son had toddled up to me, clearly tired. So I nursed him to sleep and forgot about my predicament momentarily. He had just fallen into a deep sleep when I *finally, joyously* felt the first significant jab of pain. YES! That really was my reaction. I was so happy and relieved and I just *knew* this time it was the real deal. I happily jumped out of bed and went off to time my contractions and be alone with my breath for a little while. My mood had changed completely, I was now excited and focused as I slipped into my 'warrioress' suit and mindset. Two minutes, two minutes, two minutes, very consistent pattern. How exciting. How wonderful. Time to call the midwife. It was late at night by now. She might be sleeping. But guess what? That's the beauty of it. It was great to call up my now friend and have her come over within minutes, no more guilt, no more worries about how she may have been asleep or was busy with another patient. She was there to be with me and this time around I was really okay with that. Turns out she wasn't asleep anyways. She said she had a feeling that I would be calling her that night and was waiting up to hear from me.

Thank God I forgot to give any more thought to my stomach muscles. For some reason that I have never been able to determine, as soon as my labour started, 'poof' no more muscle pain. Was it the adrenaline? The oxytocin? Divine intervention? I really have no idea. One minute I could barely move my body without it hurting and the next the pain was gone.

My eldest daughter was having trouble settling into sleep, so I decided to lay next to her to see if I could help put her down faster. As I laid on my side I experienced my first, only and last strong contraction on my back. No frigging way. The pain shot up from a 4 to a 10 suddenly and I almost felt like I couldn't navigate through it. No way could I lie down and go through contractions. So plan #2 was put into motion and we had someone we trusted come over to sit with our daughter, basically watching movies and keeping her (hopefully) pre-occupied while I got on with the baby business.

In the end she never went to sleep. Thankfully my one-year-old son had already done so. But would he stay asleep? I needed things to progress quickly. It was late at night and they would only go so long without needing my attention at that young age. We didn't have anywhere else we were comfortable sending them yet, and still I could not afford to be distracted from the birthing.

Tanya, our midwife, and my partner set everything up and gave me the space to just keep walking, pacing, and massaging the backs of my wrists and forearms, (using pressure points to encourage the labour). I was listening to some music by Snatam Kaur, one of my favourite artists, and meditating to the words while I walked. The candles were lit and lights dimmed. I was gradually and progressively gathering my nerves together for what was to come. Whenever I had to pause to answer a question or use the bathroom, I would feel the fear come swarming back and doubts creep in. I had to mentally shake myself out of it before any panic could sink in. What if this took too long, what if I couldn't manage the pain, what if, what if, what if? I thanked the fear and then shoved it away and went back to my pacing and breathing in solitude.

I intuitively knew this labour was going to be the fastest one yet. It was also significantly easier to navigate and especially much less overwhelming than the first labour. I was surprised by how much longer I was able to stay walking around during this labour compared to the previous ones.

I kept walking slowly and breathing for what seemed like a long time (in reality it wasn't) and had almost started to wonder if the baby was actually coming when my mood shifted and I felt the need to settle more and get more grounded. No more opening bags or boxes around me. No one talking. Gently rub my back and everyone stay nice and quiet. Please and thank you. I was easily able to verbally describe what I was feeling, where the baby was positioned and to signal how fast the contractions were coming.

The final stages came and went pretty quickly. I felt that the baby was just about ready to be born when my attention was diverted. Our babysitter upstairs wanted to know when she could leave so she could go home and attend to her own child. This put a strain on my hubby who was running up and down the stairs trying to answer questions. Mercifully, he decided to keep me out of the discussion of 'how long it would be.'

A few minutes later I got sucked into an overwhelming feeling of complete powerlessness, my body was 100% doing its own thing and I was helpless and glued to the spot, holding onto my breath like a lifeline, breathing as slowly and as deeply as I could over and over, eyes closed, staying present with the feelings inside. The urge to push came on suddenly, coupled with a crazy painful and scary feeling as the baby proceeded to drop through and out. I thought about resisting this feeling, there was suddenly so much pressure internally I felt total fear that I would be internally injured long-term, but then I completely let go. I clearly remember the feeling of physically and mentally deciding to just accept the situation, surrendering totally as I dropped the fight completely. One push and one split second later the little darling was born, 'en caul,' without even a squeak. (En caul means she was born still inside her amniotic sac, which occurs only once in about every 80,000 births, and is said to be considered a very lucky sign). I was delighted and scooped her up immediately and held her to my chest. It felt wonderful to hold her, to learn she was a girl, and to be done with the whole ordeal.

It was a blue moon, a full moon, and a beautiful summer night. This baby seemed to just radiate joy and peacefulness so we eventually gave her the middle names of Luna and Shanti. After we weighed her (she was not to be outdone, and although she *looked* slighter, she weighed exactly the same amount, no exaggeration, as her siblings at birth, almost 9 pounds) and took care of the other details we all snuggled up on the couch.

It was so nice to be home, so cool to have her siblings be present to say hello (even though the movie watching was much more interesting than the little baby). I was overjoyed to contact my friends and family and share the moment. I stayed up most of the remaining night writing to people to share the news. Once again a sense of joy and accomplishment raced through me. I had this healthy little angel beside me and just felt that everything would be 'okay,' at least for the time being. Tanya was wonderful and told me I should share with others whatever it was I had just done (the focus, the breathing, the meditation, etc.). I was flattered and humbled. It's hard to describe the rush of confidence that comes after this type of experience. It's not a cocky feeling, it's more like, holy crap, I just finished the marathon!!

The next day I ordered a favourite breakfast in bed and gave myself permission to enjoy the chocolate bars my dad brought me when friends and family came to visit. My team of midwives came to check on me as is status quo. I felt great physically except for my insanely sore stomach muscle. The pain was suddenly back and I couldn't even sit up without help for a day or two. I saw my osteopath several days after the birth. After she checked the baby over and did some gentle craniosacral therapy on her she gently worked on my lower abdomen. I could still barely move about and she told me I had a tear in my deep transverse abdominal tissue and that I needed to take it very seriously. My treatment plan was to do pretty much nothing, especially any exercises that taxed the core, for at least two full weeks while it healed, or else!

For at least the next little while I was able to bask in the glow of the afterbirth and rejoice in my latest family member. I now had three children under 4 years of age and we all snuggled up and stayed close throughout the first days while I took it easy. Pressure from the work world this time around meant that rather quickly it was just me and the three little kids. At first I worried about how on earth to mother all three at once, especially since they were so very young. My very first outing with all three of them, one newborn and two toddlers, brought on a wild 'holy crap is this even technically safe?' type of feeling. It was a little overwhelming to think I was totally responsible for all three. Bit-by-bit, day-by-day, I tested my courage and grew my parenting muscles. Like everything else it just took practice, willpower and patience.

Home Birth

Pain Management

"You will forget all about it once it's done. And your body will give you the hormones you need to help you through it."

"This still doesn't make me feel better."

"You can do this. Many millions have done it before you so why not you? There is certainly nothing special about you."

"Very funny."

"Thank you. I try."

You know, I really wish I could sit here and say what an awe-inspiring, amazing, incredible and *comfortable* process birth was. And it was all those things, of course it was. Except the comfortable part. Garbage and nonsense. At least for me. Emotionally and mentally maybe so, but even then, limits got tested, again and again. You think you had endurance beforehand? Wow! I had read and intuitively figured that the female body *is* able to handle pain and to get through a labour. I understood this conceptually but would have to go through labour three times to really feel the truth of this. I remember thinking, when things heated up the first time around, *I can't do this.* Well, I didn't do it. My body did. Nothing else on the outside was able to save me from the pain or the process. I had to do it and I found what I needed to get through it from within, not from without.

To me, the pain of birth is more functional and even somehow more organized, and had a more logical purpose to it. Although it seemed counter-intuitive to go head-first and completely surrender to something that was at moments (I'm not going to BS here by sugar coating) *seriously f-ing painful,* especially the first time around, I realized that was what, in fact, I had to do. By the time my third pregnancy reached its final stages I was still very scared of the pain of birth but also ready to look it straight in the eye, even hold its hand. It was like we proceeded together as a unit at that point. My pain told me what to do and where I was at in the process. Sometimes I wondered if it was tricking me (was the baby *really* about to come?) but overall it was a pretty steady and consistent birth partner.

Those beautiful birthing tubs, ready for warm water, ready to relax my weary muscles and mind. We didn't use them even once. I was, however, very comforted knowing that the tubs were at our disposable, just in case. Turns out I would be more comfortable on dry land, either walking around or with my head buried in some comfy pillows.

I didn't want or need the TENS (transcutaneous electrical nerve stimulation) unit either. When it came down to it I didn't want anything much to distract me from my mission (although psychologically I was happy to know these supportive tools were nearby, just in case). I needed to relax into the natural process of birth and to trust that the body knows what to do. Secondly, I needed a clean house and someone trusted and close to the family to watch and entertain my children. I also needed open space to move around. A solid partner by my side for support. Low lighting and relaxing, very soothing uplifting music. The reassurance of my midwives nearby, but not constantly in my personal space. Silence and stillness from those around me. Being able to feel safe and secure so that I could focus on absolutely nothing but allowing my body to go through its own process, head on. I needed to feel my environment was very peaceful and calm so that I could pull out my warrior side, throw my backpack of courage over my shoulder, tuck my still sometimes terrified little inner child into my breast pocket, and FOCUS. Doing this was far from easy, but I had my tools ready to help me walk through it. I am described sometimes as being 'spiritual,' yet when it came time to give birth I proceeded very logically and pragmatically. I let my body be as bossy as possible. Whatever made the body comfortable (pacing, dancing, hugging, hip circles, swaying, walking meditation) I did it.

I found that during the active stages of labour

the slightest unexpected sound was distracting and frankly annoying as it would pull me out of relaxation and my patterned slow breathing. On some level during birth I actually felt *guilty* for having these lovely women sit by with nothing much to do while I laboured. I genuinely felt concerned that they would be bored, or hungry, or even ignored (I know, I know, people pleasing issues. I am working on it!).

I remember at one point during birth number three my midwife was taking what seemed like a very long time in setting up the standard home birthing equipment (basically what you would see in a level one hospital room) which involved all sorts of packages being opened. I barely recognized the kitchen once she was done, as there were medical supplies, birth accessories and paperwork neatly placed pretty much everywhere. I had thought she was finished setting up and could finally relax into the silence when I heard yet one more plastic package being ripped open. It made me snap and I felt a little awkward asking her to hold the silence for the time being. Tanya was a trooper and didn't take anything personally of course. I think she actually smiled. I suspected she may have just been trying to keep busy as she had nothing else to do at that point. I don't think she knew exactly what to do with me, or what to expect from me, someone who basically asked to be left alone (except for heart rate checks) until literally the last minute. When it was time to expel the baby my body would just let go and did so without any sort of direction from me. I just kept concentrating on breathing in a very slow and steady way.

I think the most important tool I had, and the one thing I could control, was my breath. Over and over I remember taking these focused breaths and trying to slow them down, as my body clawed its way through the more painful contractions; it sort of felt like a complete animal-self coming through. I would move with the breath if needed and/or vocalize, though for the most part I was pretty silent, conserving my energy. Not running away from the pain was by no means easy to do. Sounds obvious? Nope, not really. I found that labour was like being slapped upside the head during a big storm from every possible direction, over and over *and over* again. I couldn't afford to hold my breath or to tense up my muscles. I cannot stress this point enough. When some labour pains were overwhelming and threatened to throw me off course, my ability to stay the course during each breath was paramount. Long deep breaths became my friend and lighthouse.

Of course, I had more than one friend. Pain and fear were always there, married together it seemed. The deeper the pain the more I was afraid it would get even worse or that I just "couldn't handle it." I understand now that the pain is there as a guidepost, to tell me when to breathe, when to relax, and to shuffle me along the way, to let me know how close I am to the end. And some days that even gives me a touch of belated encouragement. Even though I resented the heck out of it at the time, I can somewhat appreciate its important role. But no, I don't see it as a flowery blessing. Pain sucks. It's brutal. It feels like punishment. But there *are* things that can help. Now I can also appreciate the role of fear as well. It was making sure I paid attention, and that I stayed present and didn't focus on anything else.

Surprisingly, this breathing technique I used throughout labour, commonly referred to as bhastrika breath, came to me mostly of my own accord. I know this is taught in certain birth preparation classes. However, beyond that, it was interesting that no one at all talked to me about how to breathe throughout the *entire* length of labour, even when I would ask point blank for tips. I mostly felt that people didn't want to prescribe or tell me what to do. Fair enough. People would simply tell me to 'remember to breathe' when I asked what I should do. But remember to breathe *how* exactly? I do not think it's simply natural or obvious. When shit hits the fan I like to have something to hold onto, something I can actually *do* to help, and this became second nature.

The flip side from feeling anxiety before birth, to the fear and pain of giving birth, to the elation of accomplishing it, is such an interesting enigma.

Over and over I remember how I kept earnestly trying to bring my attention back to my body even though that was the last place where I wanted it to be once a contraction hit! This was by no means easy to do. My midwife had told me that true labour would take 100% of my concentration, it would pull me away from everything else with its intensity. Boy was she right. I remember it being very much a paradox, forcing myself to dive head first, over and over, into a rather painful sensation, when my mind was very much wanting me to do anything but! As labour progressed I just wanted out, to be anywhere but paying attention to how my body was feeling, to escape into some fanciful dreamland somewhere, to really not be experiencing what I was experiencing. When I would get distracted I would remind myself that not paying attention would only slow things down.

Gradually I started sharing what I had experienced with my own students in pre-natal yoga classes. Not long afterwards I received a letter from a pre-natal student who had been very dedicated and sometimes stayed after class to learn more. She was brand new to yoga and meditation and was planning a hospital birth with her doctor. As the business of life crept in once the class had ended we lost touch. She eventually wrote to tell me that her hospital birth had gone very well, and she gave full credit to everything she had learned in the yoga class. No fuss, no meds, she'd been focused on breathing and had felt confidently in charge and it had gone quicker than she'd hoped. I was touched she'd shared her story with me and still wish we had kept in touch longer term.

It is a little strange to say that 'just breathe through it' is probably my biggest tip for birth. I cringe at how simple and even cocky or dismissive it sounds. I think one of the secrets is in *how* you do so, and are you *set up comfortably to* do so, and are the people around you *giving you what you need* in order to be able to do so? With home birth you study, you learn a lot, you make a plan and then you make several alternative plans as back up (and yes you need them, it happens). You feel fear and also independence. In the end, wherever you give birth, there is prep work that can be done psychologically and physically. I've tried to outline most of the things I've learned and used but I am sure there are many, many other tools out there not widely shared, yet.

Final Thoughts, for Now...

An in-law of mine, someone who was once very close to me, once joked out loud after hearing about my third natural birth at home, that I was 'a freak of nature.' Or maybe he wasn't joking at all. No matter. But I assure you I am not. I am not the first woman to have an at-home birth or an unassisted birth or a birth without pain meds, and I am certainly not the first young woman to use the birthing techniques that I did.

I am of the view that there is nothing much different about me. I looked for information and a health provider who 'fit' during a very vulnerable time in my life. I had to face a huge undertaking and had to figure out what I needed to know to get us both (baby and mom) through. When I was pregnant I couldn't find books on personal home birth experiences or non-medical birth memoirs in general. There was so much I knew so little about when first embarking on this journey and many, many of my opinions got flipped on their heads.

As much as I wanted to, birth is not something I could control, and that was not easy to come to terms with. Many teachers and authors have spoken about the ability of the body to do what's best and this process really brought that home for me in a concrete way. But still in the end it was not me in control. The biggest thing I learned was to surrender. To the unknown, to the wisdom of the body and the experience and knowledge of the team of midwives supporting me.

What I liked most about having client-centred care providers on my team was that all planning efforts always considered multiple components of my health and my needs, not theirs. We planned around what worked best for me and my baby and not vice-versa. With midwives I felt like a trusted partner, whose knowledge of my own body was taken seriously. I felt like I climbed a bloody mountain barefoot and returned with a new sense of resilience like nothing before, all the while being cheered on by a supportive group of women.

Looking back with a bird's-eye view on birth, I wouldn't change anything even if I could. Mostly I am like a tea bag steeped in gratitude. And tons of it. If some of this experience lends itself to helping other women even better. The process of birth and becoming a parent has enormously added to my self-knowledge; my limits, my hidden judgments and truths, my deepest fears and my greatest strengths. I believe my experiences happened as they did largely because the team I chose to work with allowed me my own autonomy when I asked for it. Being pregnant was the one time in my life I had to rise up to my fullest stature and hold my ground, to dig deep and root my position into the ground and be firm on what I really felt was best for me and my body. The team I had around me enabled me to do that.

While I did not hire a doula for my home births, I certainly did consider it more than once. I have heard from others how this supportive service can be very helpful, reassuring and beneficial to a peaceful birth process. In my opinion both doulas and midwives are like strong warriors, willing to jump into the unknown over and over again and hold the hand of women in their most challenging moments. They risk being a witness to things going wrong and to things going right, they risk feeling scared and powerless, they risk having their hearts broken with compassion and joy every day at work, and they bravely stare down and agitate to remove the historical stigma and dogma that says a birth should be done 'status quo.' They work to change the status quo. I cannot imagine this to be an 'easy' job, no matter how rewarding it might be. Brave souls indeed.

I was fascinated by the idea that someone is willing to venture into the birthing space over and over again. It's beautiful, it's transformational, it's unpredictable, it's scary. Having had the honour of supporting a very close friend through a recent birth (in a hospital), I understand just what a privilege it is! I asked my beautiful friend who has worked for years as a doula and has witnessed many births, to share her perspectives on having a role like this. I also asked her what needs to be in place to make things easier for women in labour:

"I would describe helping women through birth at home as being an honour. Witnessing the primal instincts of any birthing mother is an honour, but allowing birth to unfold with minimum interruption is powerful! I agree that women are like an ecosystem, there is no one-size-fits-all solution as each woman is unique and needs to be heard, respected, and allowed to walk her own birthing journey.

It is hard to generalize because every healthcare provider is different, however the main difference I have experienced between midwife supported births and other births is that most midwives are aware of and most importantly respect the physiological changes in a birthing woman (however I have seen doctors do that as well, and midwives who do not - usually the ones who work from an approach based on fear). These are the changes that happen in a woman's body and her mind to prepare her for the delivery and they cannot be rushed. There are the obvious physical changes, such as the baby moving downwards, the pelvis gradually opening up and the lower spine of the woman moving backward (This last is known as the rhombus of Michaelis, and being on one's back can prevent this important shift in a mother's spine).

There is also the need of mothers to feel grounded and stable. Even if they are not standing during labour there is usually a need to put their feet on something to allow women to feel this sense of stabilization. Women also need quiet because they need to focus inwards. Darker and smaller, less open spaces without big glaring lights help birthing women feel safer and to relax and open to the process. Midwives know the importance of allowing the body to do whatever it needs to do to give birth. For example, vocalization, breath-work, meditation, using mantras, or chanting or staying absolutely quiet. Women have a choice to either concentrate on the pain and discomfort or to concentrate on the breath. Breath allows the energy to move downwards whereas fear raises it upwards. You cannot deliver through your head, you have to deliver through your body. If you are stuck in thinking mode you cannot deliver your baby as easily. The breath reminds us to stay focused on the body.

Overall the most important things a woman needs to progress well in labour are love, patience, to be uninterrupted, and an environment a woman considers calming and safe. This is most often within quiet, calm, dark surroundings with pleasant smells and sounds and carefully chosen people to love them and give them a hand when needed. What pregnant women in this modern world most need is to believe in themselves, to trust their bodies, and to be supported to feel in control of their birthing decisions without fear of judgement."

- Zoia

I am not totally biased. My style and choices certainly wouldn't suit everyone as birth is certainly not a one-size-fits-all situation. Not everyone is going to feel safe in the same space or in the same way. What I would really like to do here is encourage more discussion about the needs of women and their babies at a very special and sensitive time in their lives. *It's the having of the conversation in the first place that I feel is most important here.* I think we women are like ecosystems, all parts of our lives and environment interplay and are interdependent on one another, and we can therefore benefit from a holistic approach to birth preparation, where we tailor the needs to the individual.

I see so many instances now where I once took for granted that someone else knew what was best for me. I started this journey afraid I had lost my power and capacity to decide things. In our society we generally associate power with knowledge. More to the point, we often view whomever is in power as having the most knowledge on a subject. Digging a little deeper I hit an important question: what exactly is 'knowledge' anyways? What gets constituted as valid? And is the knowledge I need to make the right choice even written down? Or is it simply passed on orally from one woman to the next?

Do I know something is right because someone else told me so, because a study was done or because it just feels right to me? To me there are no right answers. These are just questions I have toyed with while I pondered how best to move forward making choices. Do I listen to the experts, and if so which expert, or do I listen to my own instincts? Can I become my own expert and can I somehow create a path that allows me to do both?

When it comes to pregnancy and birthing I have seen there are power struggles and cultural fluctuations and greatly different belief systems at play. I wish to encourage a new dialogue on how we can approach being pregnant and giving birth, as a society. I say being informed every step of the way is key. There is a *wealth* of information and knowledge that exists outside of the traditional western paradigm, midwifery included. It is slowly becoming more mainstream, is backed by science, and there are existing studies to prove it is safe according to specific quantitative methodology. I think it's basically like getting an invitation to be the leader of your own journey, and I appreciated the experience such that I am happy to recommend it to others.

In the end I put on my big girl undergarments and went with myself as the expert on knowing the strengths and limitations of my body, my mind and my nervous system. I decided to be the expert on where and under what circumstances I would be the most or least stressed out. It took some experimentation and it wasn't perfect but I can totally live with the results. I still smile to think that many of the old-fashioned techniques and concepts I used for PMS are the same ones that pulled me through labour.

To the Fathers

My old friend John looks up at me. He looks different today. Of course. He just had his first baby, and this is a big time in his life. I am excited for him and want to hear about how it all went. I haven't had children yet. I want to eventually but am still gathering my nerve and wits to do so at that point. I can tell he is more shaky, more excited, more raw than usual. He tells me all is well and he now has a beautiful baby girl. They had a team of supportive midwives. Mom is doing okay now and he is able to go back to work feeling mostly guilt free for leaving the two of them at home. I gently pry a little more, terribly interested in the subject matter and hoping for some more personal details. I don't want the glossy, sanitized version. I want to know what it's really like. He trusts me and is very willing to share. Suddenly he looks afraid, shaky and nervous. All I can do is offer what I have, so he readily accepts my hug and seems to hang on as though he can't let go. I realize the impact this has had on him is great and really sense how he truly experienced whatever happened alongside his wife.

"Cera, I was sooo scared." It seems to take a toll on him to admit this to me, as though it brings him right back into the moment. The moment, he tells me, he 'felt-so-helpless.' He is near tears, and suddenly so am I. His fear and memory of feeling powerless as he speaks is palpable and deeply moves me. He tells me how at the

171

very end things slowed down, his wife became exhausted and had little left to give. There is a serious debate over whether to use some vacuum or forceps intervention or to give it some more time to progress. Team A doesn't want to chance the physical and long-term developmental risks to the baby and the potential damage for mom. Team B says they had better do it anyways. My friend tells me he helplessly stands to the side holding her hand and just wills his wife and baby to make it through okay.

When the baby is finally born he is on his knees with gratitude, and still is today.

Lest I make it sound like this was a totally solo journey, it wasn't. I had support not only from my midwives but from an awesome partner, all along the long winding painfully slow road. I had a hand to hold and arms to cry in and someone to massage my feet when I was at my absolute worst. I am lucky and beyond grateful to the open-minded person in my life who was open enough to read birthing books and watch videos alongside me and rub my back while I experienced the hardest event of my life. I always knew he was there, steady, consistent and calm, and I know his supportive energy was a large part of accomplishing what I did. Many of my closest friends these days who also go through similar birthing situations also speak of the tremendous, often unrecognized support of their mates. We women get all the spotlight, which seems only fair since we go through the transformation, yet we are only as strong as the support system beneath us. To all fathers and to all the partners who have gone unrecognized I salute you and publicly thank you. Birth is not just a woman thing, it's a people thing.

Home Birth

A New Chapter, A New Outlook

I feel that fear tries to stop us from trying new ways of doing things in order to keep us safe. Fear was behind a lot of my judgments going into this journey. I never, ever would have thought I would be someone who would have a home birth. EVER. It made such a difference to consider different paths before making up my mind, instead of being told what to do or what would happen. Despite all the evidence I had accumulated over my life to the contrary, something new and different was possible after all.

I hope this story might be seen as an invitation to take a breath, no matter what birthing environment we find ourselves in. I wrote this book because I love to see women and their support teams empowering each other and encouraging each other to do whatever they need to do in order to feel healthy and safe as mothers. I love it when I hear about a mother's dignity and personal integrity being kept intact even when her plans went haywire or she was forced into a birthing path she did not choose. I am encouraged when I hear people sharing practical advice on universal subjects, even those that make us cringe and blush, like what positions for delivery put the least pressure on your pelvic floor or how to do pelvic floor exercises properly before and afterwards to avoid long-term incontinence.

Simply, I created a new narrative for myself that wasn't fear-based, integrating the suggestions from some incredibly knowledgeable, open-minded and brave teachers who didn't beat around the bush. In many ways putting it altogether and writing this memoir has been a labour of love (pun intended), and a self-growth journey on its own. I want to offer a gentle hand to hold for any women who are afraid of childbirth or pregnancy. I have been there. I did not master this fear, but I did learn to dance with it, each of us taking turns as the lead partner. Birthing this book has been a whopper, and I almost backed out of it here and there: fear of pain, feeling powerless, being misunderstood, being embarrassed and condemnation from others for preachiness or privilege, so many 'what ifs' raced through my mind as I came close to finishing it that I reached a point where I almost walked away from the project cold turkey. Almost. And that is what labour is like to me, feeling the fear, and staying on your path anyways.

Hands down, walking directly into childbirth, super scared yet steady, hand-holding my fear gently, and then straight out the other side, has given me courage I never imagined possible. Fear is more like a well-meaning friend who means only to protect me, to warn me. I am learning to love this friend but certainly not let it rule my life. Feel it, breathe it, thank it, and go forward anyways. My sister always likes to say that we should do something each day that scares us. I think of that each time I don't know how to get through tense parenting moments or when I am worried a new routine or idea will fall flat in front of my students. Is it really, perhaps, just like a muscle that gets stronger with use?

I'm forever learning to dance in the middle of a complex storm each day, every day, as I navigate parenting work and housework and 'work-work' and teaching (which rarely feels like work-work since I enjoy it so much). Unknowns and uncertainties are around every corner, despite the insanely rewarding moments. I am grateful for access to choices and information as I strive to trust my own instincts while carving a unique, tailored mothering path. It's not easy. It's no joke. May the conversation continue and each parent find a hand to hold.

Cera Gagnon loves to hear from readers.
To continue the conversation, ask questions or learn more please contact her via:

E-mail:
info@thefunfitnessgroup.com

Facebook:
https://www.facebook.com/homebirthmemoir